Medical Terminology

GENEVIEVE LOVE SMITH
PHYLLIS E. DAVIS

Medical Terminology
A PROGRAMMED TEXT
5th Ed.

Revised by

Jean Tannis Dennerll, B.S., CMA

Coordinator, Medical Assistant Program
Jackson Community College
Jackson, Michigan

A Wiley Medical Publication

JOHN WILEY & SONS, INC.
NEW YORK / CHICHESTER / BRISBANE / TORONTO / SINGAPORE

Library of Congress Cataloging in Publication Data:

Smith, Genevieve Love.
  Medical terminology.

  (A Wiley medical publication)
  Includes bibliographies and index.
  1. Medicine—Terminology—Programmed instruction.
I. Davis, Phyllis E. II. Dennerll, Jean Tannis.
III. Title. IV. Series. [DNLM: 1. Nomenclature—
programmed instruction. W 18 S648m]

R123.S6 1988   610′.14   87-13292
ISBN 0-471-83644-3 (pbk.)

Printed in the United States of America

10 9 8 7 6 5 4 3 2 1

PREFACE TO THE FIFTH EDITION

Medical Terminology: A Programmed Text, 5th Edition, is a basic text teaching a word building system for defining, using, spelling, and pronouncing medical words. Thousands of words may be built from learning the Latin and Greek word parts. The word building system, as developed by Genevieve Smith and Phyllis Davis and refined through four editions of *Medical Terminology: A Programmed Text,* continues to be an accessible and successful means for individuals and groups to learn medical terminology quickly and easily. In the 10 years I have been teaching medical terminology I have been amazed by the successful results using this text. The programmed approach with review sheets, as well as the audiotapes and tests that accompany *Medical Terminology,* provide an excellent opportunity for mastery with little or no previous study in the health care field required.

I am excited to present the new and revised features offered by this fifth edition of *Medical Terminology:*

1. Many terms are presented in new locations and grouped by subject areas. For example, all the female reproductive system terms are introduced in the same section. Words still appear in several places consistent with the programmed learning model for review and to enhance recall.

2. New, revised, and more detailed illustrations are included with special labeling of combining forms next to many anatomic terms.

3. Detailed, expanded medical abbreviation lists have been created in Appendix C. These more comprehensive lists reflect newly developed medical technology and are grouped by the following six subject areas: weights and measures, chemical symbols, diagnoses, procedures, health professions, and charting.

4. Case studies are new to this edition and have been included near appropriate words and subjects. These case studies demonstrate contextual use of medical terms and abbreviations, enrich vocabulary with additional terms not found in frames, provide an opportunity to use the word-building system to decipher meanings of unfamiliar terms, and are useful for review of terms previously presented. These reports were condensed from actual cases provided by the Medical Records Department at W. A. Foote Memorial Hospital in Jackson, Michigan.

5. Several new frames have been added to update the text, and obsolete or redundant frames have been deleted. The most up-to-date lists of medical diagnoses and procedures are found in the International Classification of Diseases, 9th edition, Clinical Modification (ICD-9-CM) and Current Procedural Terminology (CPT) code books, and these books have been used to determine the content of this fifth edition.

6. The Review Sheets are revised to reflect the changes in the text and their corresponding frame numbers are added for ease of reference.

7. The ancillary materials, useful for teaching groups, have been updated and revised. These include audiotapes as well as the instructor's manual, which provides suggestions for teaching, completely revised and expanded tests, crossword puzzles, and additional case studies. These materials, while useful to the instructor, are supplementary to the text. Any student may successfully learn from the text itself without these materials.

I gratefully acknowledge the people who gave their support and assistance in the preparation of this fifth edition of *Medical Terminology.* I especially thank my husband and computer specialist, Timothy J. Dennerll; my mother and child care giver, Helen Tannis; my sister and typist, Arlene Tannis Coward; my colleagues at Jackson Community College; my mentor and editor, Jane de Groot; illustrator Kitty Herman; and the gracious staff of John Wiley & Sons, Inc.

I also acknowledge the many students, instructors, and professional staff who tested and offered constructive suggestions for the fifth edition. I thank Diane Jonas, Medical Transcription Supervisor, W. A. Foote Memorial Hospital, Jackson, Michigan, for her assistance in the preparation of the case studies.

It is my intention that *Medical Terminology: A Programmed Text,* 5th Edition, continue the success and traditional integrity of this classic text.

Jean Tannis Dennerll, B.S., CMA

PREFACE TO THE FOURTH EDITION

The three previous editions of this book were well received and widely used. That the text successfully met the tests of use is no accident. The original text was developed in the classroom from a list of medical terms. In the five years preceding publication of the first edition, the effectiveness of content, organization, and frame structures were tested against student responses. During that period of time the text was actually revised no fewer than seven times. Refinement of the text continued in the classroom through 1969, two years after the second edition had met widespread acceptance. Since then, helpful suggestions from teachers, the formats of foreign translations, reviews by professionals, students' comments, and continued research have kept the book alive and well.

In presenting this fourth edition of *Medical Terminology,* the authors wish to emphasize the improvements that have been made in this revision. They are in four main areas:

1. The most extensive improvement has been made in the pronunciation system. It has been completely revised in the fourth edition. The ideal pronunciation system represents each significant sound with one and only one symbol. Although no system is perfect, we think that our new system, which utilizes a few simple diacritics and the schwa (ə), is much more accurate than the old one. Anyone who uses a modern dictionary will be familiar with these symbols. A complete pronunciation key may be found on page xiii.

The new pronunciations also give greater recognition to different pronunciations of the same word, such as those for "gynecology." In this case, as in many others, two pronunciations (jin · ə · kol′ə · jé and gi · nə · kol′ə · je) are both widely used and equally acceptable. We cannot, however, give all regional variations, as in the pronunciation of terms like "human," which is pronounced hyoo′mən or yoo′mən, depending upon the region in which one resides. One will, naturally, adopt the pronunciations of one's locality. But the simplicity of the system and its consistency throughout should certainly be a great aid to the beginning student of medical terminology.

2. The index is an addition of considerable importance to the text. This complete index, locating all terms taught by the text, should make it much easier for the student to look up a term when the need arises.

3. New illustrations have been added to heighten interest and further reinforce the significance of terms, particularly in relation to anatomy.

4. Alterations and modernizations have been made in 87 frames, and 28 completely new frames have been inserted to replace obscure, ineffective, or obsolete frames.

The need for the text remains as pressing today as it was when the first edition was published. Newcomers to the health field still think of the language of medicine as an almost insurmountable obstacle. The objective of the text remains to make the terminology of medicine understandable as well as easy, even fun, to learn. The methods of the programmed text also remain unchanged, and the evidence of their effectiveness continues to be strong.

Medical terminology is a technically exact vocabulary used by professionals to speak and write precisely. Most terms are compound words consisting of joined Greek or Latin word roots, combining forms, prefixes, and suffixes. The meanings of the component parts are understood through that branch of the study of languages known as etymology. Etymology is not an unfailing guide to a word's meaning or to all it may connote, but it does furnish valuable insights. This text exploits those insights.

The meanings of word parts, a word-building system based on these parts, and the programmed teaching technique are combined in this text to:

1. furnish an understanding of the need and reason for the technical language of medicine.
2. demonstrate how terms come to be, how they are formed.
3. build a background vocabulary in medical terminology.
4. teach a complete word-building system that makes it easy for the user to understand a growing medical terminology.

The organization of the text remains unchanged. Although anatomy is said to be "the *sine qua non* for entry into fields of human biology," word parts in the text are not classified under anatomic systems. All prefixes and suffixes cut across anatomic systems, as do many combining forms, e.g., path/o, plast/o, micr/o, and troph/o. Many more word parts are used in several systems than are employed in one system only.

Other outstanding features of the book have been retained. Appendix B remains as a glossary of word parts that the student has studied in the frames. Appendix C introduces word parts that are common in medical usage but are not taught specifically in the text. This appendix, as well as other aids, should be used by teachers to help teach terms in addition to those developed in the frames. Whether or not the text is employed for self-instruction, the student will find a good dictionary to be of great aid. The new terms have, of course, been added to both appendices. The Review Sheets have been updated and are still a part of the book, to be used as required for the needs of the individual student.

The series of eight audiotapes designed to provide the student with practice in word recognition and pronunciation continues to be available. As originally intended, these tapes are to be used as a supplementary drill outside the classroom and as a review prior to administration of each of eight tests. They are also especially helpful to those who are teaching themselves medical terminology. Further information may be obtained from the publisher, John Wiley & Sons, Inc., Medical Division.

We are grateful to the many students and teachers who have sent comments and suggestions to us and to the professional reviewers who have given us constructive criticisms. We are particularly thankful for the outstanding professional work of lexi-cographers Sidney Landau, Ron Bogus, and Robert Jones, who furnished the new pronunciation system and new pronunciations for this edition. The editors of the Medical Division of John Wiley & Sons, Inc., Cathy Somer and Andrea Stingelin, made this revision possible by their continued attention and abilities to resolve the many problems of the undertaking. We hope that the users of the text will continue to give us their valued suggestions. We, in turn, will continue to try to make medical termi-nology easily understood.

Genevieve Love Smith
Phyllis E. Davis

FOR THE READER'S INFORMATION

Objectives of the Program

Upon the completion of this text, the student will be able to:

1. build literally thousands of medical words from Greek and Latin prefixes, suffixes, word roots, and combining forms.
2. recognize medical words from the Greek and Latin parts.
3. spell medical words correctly.
4. use a medical dictionary.
5. pronounce medical terms correctly.
6. recall acceptable medical abbreviations and their meanings for medical terms and phrases.

Audiences for This Book

This text is intended to assist those studying in the fields of medicine and health care. This includes future nurses, medical assistants, pre-med students, medical secretaries, medical records librarians, radiographers, ultrasonographers, medical machine transcriptionists, physical and occupational therapists, social workers, emergency medical technicians, ward secretaries, nurse aides, respiratory therapists, laboratory technicians, and others. In addition, people in the world of business who have frequent contact with the health care field will find this text useful. This text is also intended for graduates working in allied health fields who feel the need to renew or increase their medical vocabulary.

Prerequisite

High school education.

Pretests

It is assumed that pretests would be of no value with so technical a vocabulary.

PRONUNCIATION KEY

The primary stress mark (′) is placed after the syllable bearing the heavier stress or accent; the secondary stress mark (′) follows a syllable having a somewhat lighter stress, as in **com · men · da · tion** (kom′ən · dā′shən).

a	add, map	m	move, seem	u	up, done
ā	ace, rate	n	nice, tin	er	urn, term
air	care, air	ng	ring, song	yo͞o	use, few
ä	palm, father	o	odd, hot	v	vain, eve
b	bat, rub	ō	open, so	w	win, away
ch	check, catch	ô	order, jaw	y	yet, yearn
d	dog, rod	oi	oil, boy	z	zest, muse
e	end, pet	ou	out, now	zh	vision, pleasure
ē	even, tree	o͞o	pool, food	ə	the schwa, an un-
f	fit, half	oo	took, full		stressed vowel
g	go, log	p	pit, stop		representing the
h	hope, hate	r	run, poor		sound spelled
i	it, give	s	see, pass		a in *above*
ī	ice, write	sh	sure, rush		e in *sicken*
j	joy, ledge	t	talk, sit		i in *clarity*
k	cool, take	th	thin, both		o in *melon*
l	look, rule	th	this, bathe		u in *focus*

SOURCE: Slightly modified "Pronunciation Key" in *Funk & Wagnalls Standard College Dictionary*. Copyright © 1977 by Harper & Row, Publishers, Inc. Reprinted by permission of the publisher.

The schwa (ə) varies widely in quality from a sound close to the (u) in *up* to a sound close to the (i) in *it* as heard in pronunciations of such words as *ballot, custom, landed, horses.*

The (r) in final position as in *star* (stär) and before a consonant as in heart (härt) is regularly indicated in the respellings, but pronunciations without (r) are unquestionably reputable. Standard British is much like the speech of eastern New England and the lower South in this feature.

In a few words, such as *button* (but'n) and (sud'n), no vowel appears in the unstressed syllable because the (n) constitutes the whole syllable.

LIST OF ANATOMIC ILLUSTRATIONS

CONTENTS

Medical Terminology

HOW TO WORK THE PROGRAM

answer column

1

Directions: Cover the answer column with a folded piece of paper.

A frame is a piece of information plus a blank (~~Response clue~~) in which you write. All this material following the number 1 is a _____frame_____.

Check your answer by sliding down your cover paper.

frame
Now go on to Frame 2

＊ more than 1 word   ＊＊ own word

2

By checking your answer immediately, you know whether or not you are right. This immediate knowledge helps you to learn only what is _____correct_____ _____ (correct/incorrect).

Check your answer by sliding down your cover paper.

correct
Now go on to Frame 3

3

A program is a way of learning that tells you immediately when you are correct. When you work a series of frames and are certain that you are right, you are learning from a _____program_____.

Check your answer by sliding down your cover paper.

program

4

By means of a program, you can also learn at your own speed. Learning at your own speed and having immediate knowledge that you are learning correctly are both advantages of a

_____program_____.

Always check your answers immediately.

program

1

answer column	
	5 You will learn medical terminology from a program. Class will be more interesting because you will come prepared for it having worked your
program	_program_ .
	6 When you see (_____), your answer will need only one word. In the sentence, "This is a program
medical	in ___ _medical_ ___ terminology," you
one	know to use ___ _one_ ___ word.
	7 This single blank (_____) contains a clue. It is proportional to the length of the word needed. This short blank (_____) means one short word. The long blank (_____)
long	mean one ___ _long_ ___ word.
	8 Whenever you see a blank space (_____),
one	you know to write ___ _one_ ___ (one/more than one) word. You also know something about the
length	___ _length_ ___ (length/complexity) of the word.
	9 Whenever you see a star blank (*_____), your answer will require more than one word. In the sentence, "This is a programmed course in
medical terminology	* _medical terminology_ "
more than one word	your answer requires * _more than_ .
	10 In (*_____) there is no clue to the length of the words or how many words. The important thing to remember is that (*_____) means
more than one word	* _more than 1 word_ .
anything from interesting to dull (If you did not	**11** When you see a double-star blank (**_____) use your own words. In the sen-

2

tence, "I think a programmed course in medical terminology will be **_____,"

you are expected to

** _____.

12

In the sentence, "I want to go to college because (**_____)," you are

free to ** <u>use own word</u>_____.

13

Now summarize what you have learned so far:

(_____) means <u>one</u> word

(_____) gives a clue about the <u>length</u>

_____ of the word.

(*_____) means * <u>more than</u>

_____ word.

(**_____) means ** <u>own words</u>

_____ words.

14

The fact that you check your answer immediately is very important for efficient, accurate learning. Every time you fill a blank, you will ** <u>check</u>

<u>answer</u>_____.

15

When working a program, **never look ahead.** There are many reasons for this, but the important thing to learn now is

* <u>never look ahead</u>.

16

You may always look back to find something you have forgotten. You will probably have to look back, but never look <u>ahead</u>.

17

If you make even one error, look back to see where you were incorrect. Correct the error; then go on. You may always look <u>back</u>, but <u>never</u> look ahead.

Answer column (left):

answer this one, it doesn't matter.)
use own words

use own words

one

length
more than one

use own

check the answer immediately

never look ahead

ahead

back, never

3

answer column	
correct	**18** Never let an incorrect answer go uncorrected. Each time you make an error, you _correct_ it.
	19 This is a new way of learning. **This is not a test.** Remember always, this is a way of
learning	_learning_.
back correct	**20** Do not be ashamed of a mistake; this is **not** a test. If you make an error, simply look _back_ to see where you were incorrect; then _correct_ the error.
one more than one my own	**21** Summarize what you have learned about the mechanics of working a program: (_____) means _one_ word. (*_____) means * _more than_ _____ word. (**_____) means ** _own_ _____ words.
corrected back ahead learning	**22** Continue to summarize: Any error must be _corrected_. You may always look _back_. Never look _ahead_. This is not a test. It is a way of _learning_.
	23 The material to be learned in the first 94 frames is the most important part of the entire course. This teaches the **system** of word building you will use in Medical Terminology.
	24 Since the material in the first 94 frames is so important, you will learn it thoroughly before you start

4

thoroughly, well, or
anything that means
this

to build medical words. Once you understand this
material the rest is fun. Learn the first 94 frames
** ___thoughly___

___. (How?)

25

Medical Terminology is a course designed to teach
a medical vocabulary. Physicians use a medical

vocabulary or
terminology

___terminolgy vocabulary___

26

Every field of knowledge has its own particular terminology. In the field of medicine, this is a medical

terminology or
even vocabulary

___terminology___.

27

In any field of knowledge one needs a special vocabulary to speak or write exactly. Physicians, nurses,
and allied health professionals use a medical vocabulary to speak or write ___exactly___.

exactly

THE WORD-BUILDING SYSTEM

answer column

28

Medicine has a large vocabulary, but you can learn much of it by word building. When you put words together from their parts, you are _word_ building.

word

29

All words have a word root. Even ordinary, everyday words have a * _word root_ .

word root

30

The word root is the foundation of a word. Trans/port, ex/**port**, im/**port**, and sup/**port** have **port** as their * _word root_ .

word root

31

Suf/**fix**, pre/**fix**, af/**fix**, and **fix**/ation have **fix** as their * _word root_ .

word root

32

The word root in **tonsill**/itis, **tonsill**/ectomy, and **tonsill**/ar is _tonsill_ .

tonsill

33

The foundation of the word is the
* _word root_ .

word root

34

Compound words can be formed when two word roots are used to build the word. Even in ordinary English, two word roots are used to form * _compound words_ .

compound words

6

35

Sometimes the two word roots are words. They still form a compound word. Short/hand is a

* _compound words_ .

36

Short/change, short/wave, and short/stop are also

* _compound words_ .

37

Two or more word roots mean a word is a

* _compound word_ .

38

Form a compound word using the word roots, **under and age.** _underage_

39

Form a compound word from the word roots, **chicken** and **pox.** _chickenpox_

40

A combining form is a word root plus a vowel. In the word therm/o/meter, therm/o is the

* _combining form_ .

41

In the word speed/o/meter, speed/o is the

* _combining form_ .

42

In the words micr/o/scope, micr/o/film, and micr/o/be, micr/o is the

* _combining form_ .

43

The combining form of word roots is also used to build compound words. The previous examples, therm/o/meter, speed/o/meter, micr/o/scope, and micr/o/film are

* _compound words_ .

7

44

Compound words can also be formed from a **combining form** and a whole **word**. Thermometer is a compound word built from a combining form and a word. In the word therm/o/meter:

therm/o is the

* _combing form_ ;

meter is the _word_ .

45

Build a compound word from the combining form micr/o plus:

scope _micr / o / scope_

film _micr / o / film_

meter _micr / o / meter_

46

Build a compound word from the combining form hydr/o plus:

plane _hydr / o / plane_

meter _hydr / o / meter_

foil _hydr / o / foil_

47

The words you built in Frames 45 and 46 are

compound words.

48

In medical terminology, compound words are usually built from a **combining form,** a **word root,** and an **ending.** In the word micr/o/scop/ic,

micr/o is the combining form,

scop is the word root,

(ic) is the _ending_ .

adj.

49

In the word therm/o/metr/ic,

therm/o is the combining form,

8

answer column	
word root	metr is the *___wood root___,
ending	ic is the ___ending___. (adj.)

50

In the word electr/o/metr/ic,

combining form	electr/o is the *___comb. form___,
word root	metr is the *___wood root___,
ending	ic is the ___adj. (ending)___.

51

Build a word from:
    the combining form   electr/o,
    the word root   stat,
    the ending   ic.

electr/o/stat/ic   ___electr / o / stat / ic___

52

Build a word from:
    the word root   chlor,
    the combining form   hydr/o,
    the ending   ic.

hydr/o/chlor/ic   ___hydr / o / chlor / ic___

53

Build a word from:
    the ending   ide,
    the combining form   hydr/o,
    the word root   chlor.

hydr/o/chlor/ide   ___hydr / o / chlor / ide___

54

If you missed either of the last two frames, rework the program starting with Frame 48.

55

The ending that follows a word root is a suffix. You can change the meaning of a word by putting another part after it. This other part is a

suffix   ___suffix___.

9

answer column	
	56
	The suffix **er** means **one who.** The word root, port (to carry), is changed by putting **er** after it. In the
suffix	word port/er, **er** is a ___suffix___ .
	57
	In the word read/able, able changes the meaning
suffix	of read. **able** is a ___suffix___ .
	58
	Suffixes may also change the part of speech of a word. For example, nouns (naming persons, places, or things) may be changed to adjectives (descriptors) such as:

NOUN	ADJECTIVE
cyanosis	cyanotic
anemia	anemic
nerve	nervous
mucus	mucous

	59
	In the words cyan/osis, anem/ia, duoden/um, the
osis, ia, um	noun suffixes are ___osis___, ___ia___, and ___um___.
	60
	List the suffixes that make the following terms adjectives:
tic	cyano/tic
ic	anem/ic
ous	nerv/ous
al	duoden/al
ous	muc/ous
	61
	In the words planted and planting, the suffixes are
ed, ing	___ed___ and ___ing___.
	62
planted (past)	The suffixes **ed** and **ing** added to the word root **plant**
planting (present)	create verbs (parts of speech that show action). Changing the suffix also alters the tense of a verb (when the action takes place).

10

answer column	

63

Other forms of the word inject are:

injected

_____/ ed_____ past tense

injecting

_____/ ing_____ present tense

64

A prefix is a word part that goes before a word. You can change the meaning of the word by putting another part before it. This other part is a

prefix

_prefix_____.

65

The prefix **ex** means **from.** The word root, port (to carry), is changed by putting **ex** in front of it. In

prefix

the word ex/port, **ex** is a _prefix_____.

66

In the word dis/please, **dis** changes the meaning

prefix

of please, **dis** is a _prefix_____.

67

In the words im/plant, sup/plant, and trans/plant,

im, sup, trans

the prefixes are _im_, _sup_, and _trans_.

68

Before learning more, review what you have learned. The foundation of a word is a

word root

*   _word root_____.

69

The word part that is placed before a word to change

prefix

its meaning is a _prefix_____.

70

The word part that follows a word root is a

suffix

_suffix_____.

71

adjective, verb

A suffix may change a noun to an _adj._ or change the tense of a _verb_.

11

answer column	
	72 When a vowel is added to a word root, the word part that results is a * _combing form_ .
combining form	
compound word	**73** When some form of two or more word roots is used to form a word, the word formed is called a *_____ _compound word_ .

Notice the diagrammed sentence below, which illustrates the use of adjectives, nouns, and verbs.

Diagrammed sentence:

```
      adj      noun     verb        adj      noun       adj      noun
The medical assistant charted the patient's history of duodenal ulcer.
```
   subject   predicate

HOW TO STUDY MEDICAL TERMINOLOGY

74

This is a system of word building. There are exceptions to all systems. This system of word building also has ___exception___ .

exceptions

75

It is important to learn the system. It is impossible to memorize enough medical words! By using a few word parts, you can build thousands of words, if you know the ___system___ .

system

76

Although there are exceptions to this system of word building, it is important to know the

___system___ .

system

77

When you write a new word and check your answer, you will usually find the pronunciation given. Pronounce the word **out loud** and listen to what you are saying. Practice proper pronunciation by listening to the special cassette tapes prepared to accompany *Medical Terminology*, 5th edition.

78

Each new word should be pronounced **out loud** several times. This helps you to spot exceptions to the word-building ___system___ .

system

79

Pronouncing **out loud** is not much good if you don't listen to what you are saying. Always pronounce

listen

new words **out loud** and ___listen___ to what you are saying.

80

system

Saying and listening will help you spot exceptions to the word-building ___system___.

81

Saying and **listening** will do much more for you. On the following drawing, find the parts of the brain used when saying and listening. (Refer to this drawing while working the next eight frames.)

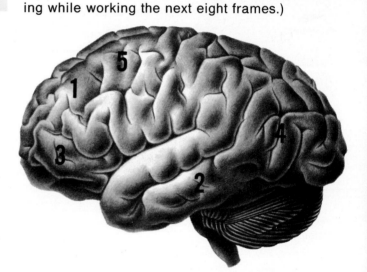

1. thinking area
2. hearing area
3. saying area
4. seeing area
5. writing area

82

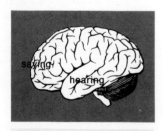

On this picture of the brain, label the parts that help you remember a word when you **say** it and **listen** to it.

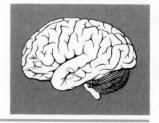

83

Do it

If you look at the word when you say it and hear it, you are using a third part of the brain to help you remember. Find the part of the brain that sees the word.

14

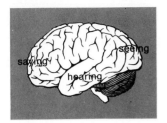

84
Label the parts of the brain that:
    say
    see
    hear

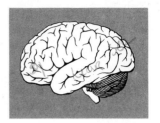

answer column
Do it

85
If you think of what you are saying, seeing, and hearing, you involve a fourth part of the brain in the memory process. Find this fourth part of the brain.

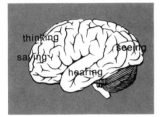

86
Label the parts of the brain that see, hear, say, and think.

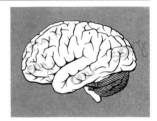

87
If you have four parts of the brain working for you at the same time, you will learn much faster. This is efficient learning. It makes sense to say a word, listen to it, look at it, and think about it in one operation.

88
Each time you see this picture you will remember to ** _____
_____
_____ .

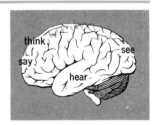

say, think, see, hear (or something that means this)

89
When you wrote the new word, you impressed it on a fifth part of the brain. Find this part of the brain on the large drawing.

See how efficiently you are learning!

90
In Appendix A there are several review sheets. You will be told when to work them and reminded to rework them. Don't worry about them now. Don't

15

ahead

even look at them, because that would be looking ___ahead___ .

91

Look at the picture in Frame 88.

You rework review sheets as soon as a word part stops **ringing in your ears.** This will be related to how well you did what the picture in Frame 88 suggests.

92

Of course, anytime you work you should ___think___ .

think

think

93

While building medical words, follow the method you have been using. If you find you are forgetting your word-building system, rework **Frames 28 through 73.**

94

While studying medical terminology, a medical dictionary is your best friend. Look up all new terms for in-depth definitions using a * ___medical dictionary___ .

medical dictionary

You are now ready to start building medical words.

MEDICAL TERMINOLOGY

answer column

95

_____A____/B_____ means a word root and its combining form. **A** is the word root; **AB** is the combining form. In acr/o, arc is the * _word root_
and acr/o is the
* _combining form_ .

word root

combining form

96

In **megal/o,** megal is the * _word root_
and megal/o is the
* _combining form_ .

word root

combining form

97

In **dermat/o,** dermat is the * _word root_
and dermat/o is the
* _combining form_ .

word root

combining form

98

acr/o
or
acr

acr/o is used to build words that refer to the extremities. To refer to extremities, physicians use words containing _acr_ .

99

acr/o is found in words concerning the extremities, which in the human body are the arms and legs. To build words about the arms use
acr /o.

acr/o

100

To build words about the legs use _acr_ /o.

acr/o

17

answer column	
	101
	acr/o any place in a word should make you think of the extremities. When you read a word containing acr or acr/o, you think of
extremities	_extremities_ .
	102
	In the word acr/o/paralysis (acroparalysis) acr/o
extremities	refers to _extremities_ .
	103
	The words acr/o/megaly (acromegaly), acr/o/ cyan/osis (acrocyanosis), and acr/o/dermat/itis (acrodermatitis) all refer to the
extremities	_extremities_ .
	104
large	**megal/o** means enlarged. Megal/o can also mean
big	large. A word containing megal/o will mean some-
enlarged	thing is ** _enlarged_ .
	105
	Acr/o/megal/y (acromegaly) means that the ex-
large, big, or enlarged	tremities are _enlarged, big_ .
	106
acr/o/megal/y	Acr/o/megal/y means enlargement of the extremi-
acromegaly	ties. The word that means a person has enlarged
ak rō meg′ ə lē	hands is _acr / o / megaly_ .
	107
	Acromegaly can be a specific disorder of the body. Symptoms are enlargement of the bones of the hands and feet, as well as some of the bones of the head. A patient with these symptoms is said to
acromegaly	have _acromegaly_ .
	108
	Occasionally you see a person with very large hands, feet, nose, and chin. The skin also has a coarse texture. This person probably has
acromegaly	_acromegaly_ .

18

answer column	
noun	**109** **y** is a suffix that makes a word a noun. Acromegaly is a ___noun___.
skin	**110** **dermat/o** refers to the skin. When you see dermat or dermat/o, think immediately of ___skin___.
skin	**111** A dermat/o/logist (dermatologist) is a specialist in a field of medicine. This person specializes in diseases of the ___skin___.
acr/o/dermat/itis acrodermatitis ak rō dûr mə tī′ tis	**112** Acr/o/dermat/itis (acrodermatitis) is a word that means inflammation of the skin of the extremities. A person with red, inflamed hands has ___acro dermatitis___.
acrodermatitis	**113** Acrodermatitis could result from stepping in a patch of poison ivy. A person with red, inflamed feet has ___acro dermatitis___.
inflammation	**114** Remembering the word acrodermatitis, which means inflammation of the skin of the extremities, draw a conclusion. **itis** is a suffix that means ___inflammed___.
cyan/o or cyan	**115** **cyan/o** is used in words to mean blue or blueness. When photographers want to say something about how a film reproduces the color blue, they use ___cyan___.
cyan	**116** Acr/o/cyan/osis means blueness of the extremities. The part of the word that tells you that the color blue is involved is ___cyan___.

19

acr/o/cyan/osis
acrocyanosis
ak rō sī ə nō′ sis

117

Acr/o/cyan/osis results from lack of oxygen. When the blood doesn't carry enough oxygen to the hands and feet, _acrocyanosis_ results.

118

When the lungs cannot get enough oxygen into the blood because of asthma, blueness of the extremities may result. This is another cause of _acrocyanosis_ .

acrocyanosis

119

osis is a suffix that makes a word a noun and means condition. To say a condition of blueness of the extremities, use the suffix _osis_ .

osis

120

Acrocyanosis is a _noun_ . (noun/verb)

noun

121

Paralysis is a word that means loss of movement. Form a compound word meaning paralysis of the extremities.

acr /o /_paralysis_

acr/o/paralysis
acroparalysis
ak rō pə ral′ ə sis

122

Dermat/itis means inflammation of the skin. The suffix that means inflammation is _itis_ .

itis

123

Dermatitis immediately forms a picture of red skin. To say that the skin is inflamed, physicians use the word _dermatitis_ .

dermat/itis
dermatitis
dûr mə tī′ tis

124

Analyze the word dermat/itis. **itis** means inflammation; **dermat** means of the _skin_ .

skin

125

Dermat/osis means any skin condition. This word denotes an abnormal skin condition. The suffix that means condition is _osis_ .

osis

20

answer column	

126

osis: is a suffix
forms a noun
means disease or condition
Build a word that means a condition of blueness.

cyan/osis
cyanosis
sī ə nō′ sis

_____cyan/osis_____

127

otic is a suffix that forms an adjective. Build the term that means pertaining to a condition of blueness.

cyan/o/tic
cyanotic
sī ə no′ tik

_____cyan/o/tic_____

128

Build a word that means condition of the skin.

dermat/osis
dermatosis
dûr mə tō′ sis

_____dermat/osis_____

129

The Greek word tomos means **a piece cut off.** From this word we have many suffixes which refer to cutting: ec/tom/y (a cutting out), o/tom/y (a cutting into), tome (an instrument that cuts). The word root for cut is _____tom_____

tom

130

Remember to associate **tom** (tome, ectomy, and otomy) with cutting. A dermatome is an instrument that cuts _____skin_____.

skin

131

A dermatome is an instrument. When a physician wants a thin slice of a patient's skin for examination under a microscope, the physician will ask for a _____dermatome_____.

dermatome
dûr′ mə tōm

132

Did you get it? If so, you are really learning medical terminology. (This one is for free.)

133

derm/o is another combining form for words referring to the skin; **pathy** is a suffix meaning disease.

21

skin

Dermopathy means a disease condition of the

Skin

---

blue skin or
bluish discoloration
of the skin
noun

134

Derma is a word itself. It is a noun meaning skin.
Cyan/o/derm/a is a compound word. It means

** *blue skin*

and is a ___*noun*___ .
(noun/adjective)

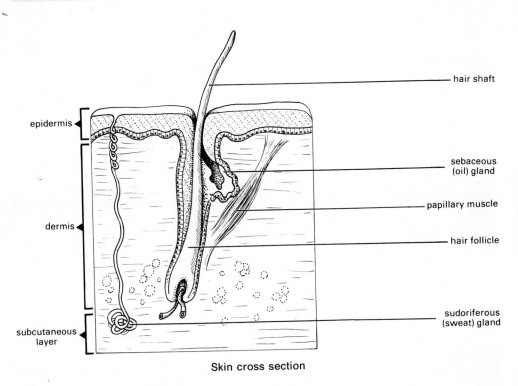

epidermis — hair shaft

dermis — sebaceous (oil) gland

— papillary muscle

— hair follicle

subcutaneous layer — sudoriferous (sweat) gland

Skin cross section

Use this information for building words involving color
(Frames 135 through 156)

leuk/o	white
melan/o	black
erythr/o	red
cyan/o	blue
chlor/o	green
xanth/o	yellow

22

135

Cyan/o/derma means blue skin. Build a word meaning:

red skin (blushing)

erythr/o/derma ;

erythr/o/derma

white skin

leuk/o/derma ;

leuk/o/derma

yellow skin

xanth/o/derma ;

xanth/o/derma

(You draw the lines)

black (discolored) skin

melan/o/derma .

melan/o/derma
(You pronounce)

136

Cyte means cell. A chlorocyte is a green cell (in plants). Build a word meaning:

black cell (dark)

melan/o/cyte

melan/o/cyte

white (blood) cell

leuk/o/cyte

leuk/o/cyte

red (blood) cell

erythr/o/cyte

erythr/o/cyte
(You pronounce)

137

Blast means embryonic cell. A leukoblast is an embryonic white cell. Build a word meaning an embryonic cell of the following color:

black

melan/o/blast

red

erythr/o/blast

melan/o/blast
erythr/o/blast
(You pronounce)

138

emia means blood. Cyan/emia is blue blood. (Not literally in people; lobsters have blue blood.) Build words involving the following colors when referring to blood conditions:

yellow xanth/emia ;

green chlor/emia ;

red (blushing) erythr/emia ;

xanth/emia
chlor/emia
erythr/emia
(You pronounce)

23

answer column	
green	
yellow	
red	
white	
black	

139

Chlor/o   means ___green___.
Xanth/o   means ___yellow___.
Erythr/o   means ___red___.
Leuk/o   means ___white___.
Melan/o   means ___black___.

---

cyan/o/derm/a
cyanoderma
sī ə nō dûr′ mə

140

Cyanoderma sometimes occurs when children swim too long in cold water. A person who has a bluish discoloration of the skin for any reason suffers from ___cyanoderma___.

---

leuk/o
or
leuk

141

leuk/o means white. There are many words in medicine that refer to white. To say something is white, use ___leuk___.

---

leuk or
leuk/o

142

In the compound word leuk/o/derm/a, the part that means white is ___leuk___.

---

white skin,
abnormally white skin,
whiteness of the skin, etc.

143

Leuk/o/derm/a means
**   ___white skin___.

---

leuk/o/derm/a
leukoderma
loo kō dûr′ mə

144

Some people have much less color in their skin than is normal. Their skin is white. They have ___leuk /o / derm / a___.

145

Some people have white areas on their skin. Sometimes these white areas are called ___leuk /o / derm / a___.

leuk/o/derm/a

146

cyt/o refers to cells. A cell is the smallest structural unit of all living things. To refer to this smallest part of the body, ___cyt / o___ is used.

cyt/o

24

answer column	
cyt/o	**147** Cytology is the study of cells. The part of cyt/o/logy that means cells is ___cyt/o___ .
cell	**148** There are several kinds of cells in blood. One kind is a leuk/o/cyt/e (refer to illustration on page 27). A leukocyte is a white blood ___cell___ .
leuk/o/cyt/e leukocyte lōō′ kō sīt	**149** There are several kinds of leukocytes in the blood. When physicians want to know how many leuko-cytes of all kinds there are, they ask for a ___leuk / o / cyt / e___ count.
leuk/o/cyt/e	**150** When physicians want to know how many there are of one kind of leukocyte, they ask for a differential ___leuk / o / cyt / e___ count.
penia	**151** Leuk/o/cyt/o/penia (leukocytopenia) means a de-crease in white blood cells. The part of the word that means **decrease in** is ___penia___ .
leuk/o/cyt/o/penia leukocytopenia lōō kō sī tō pē′ nē ə	**152** Penia is the Greek word for poverty. The word that means **decrease in** or **not enough** white blood cells is ___leuk / o / cyt / o / penia___ .
leukocytopenia	**153** If the body does not produce enough white blood cells, the patient suffers from ___leuko cytopenia___ .
leuk/em/ia leukemia lōō kē′ mē ə	**154** You have heard of leuk/em/ia, popularly called "blood cancer." ia is a noun ending. **em** comes from a Greek word meaning "blood." A noun meaning, literally, "white blood," is ___leuk / em / ia___ .

25

155

In leukemia the blood is not really white. A symptom of this disease is the presence of too many leukocytes in the blood. This symptom was used to name the disease _leukemia_.

leukemia

156

Erythr/o means red. Cells that contain a red substance (hemoglobin) are called red blood cells or _erythr/o/cytes_

erythr/o/cytes
erythrocytes
e rith′ rō sīts

157

A patient who lacks red blood cells suffers from _erthro/cyt/o/paula_

erythrocytopenia
e rith′ rō sīt ō pē′ nē ə

158

Another type of blood cell is the **thromb/o/cyte.** Thrombocytes prevent bleeding by allowing the blood to clot. An abnormal decrease in the number of these clot-forming cells is _thromb/o/cytopenia_

thrombocytopenia
thromb ō sīt ō pē nē ə

159

thromb/o means blood clot. The blood cells that cause blood clots are _thrombocytes_

thromb/o/cytes
thrombocytes
throm′ bō sīts

160

Remember, your best friend is your medical dictionary. Look up the new terms you have learned for in-depth definitions.

161

In the word acr/o/megal/y, the word root for big or large is _acr_.

megal

162

The combining form of **megal** is _megal/o_.

megal/o

163

cardi/o is the combining form for words about the heart. Cardi/o/megal/y is a noun that means ** _enlarged heart_.

large heart
enlargement of
the heart

26

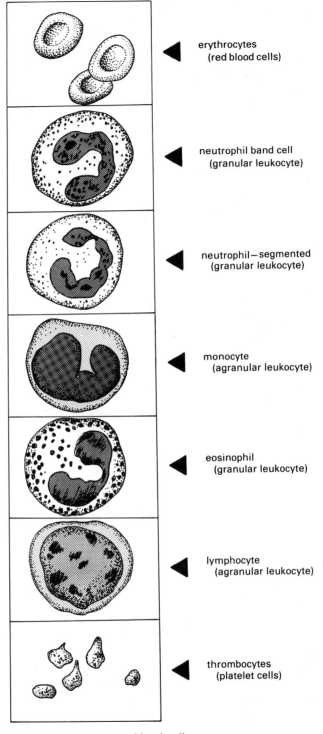

erythrocytes
(red blood cells)

neutrophil band cell
(granular leukocyte)

neutrophil—segmented
(granular leukocyte)

monocyte
(agranular leukocyte)

eosinophil
(granular leukocyte)

lymphocyte
(agranular leukocyte)

thrombocytes
(platelet cells)

blood cells

answer column	

Megal/o/cardia also means enlargement or over-development of the heart. When something causes overgrowth of the heart,

megal/o/cardi/a
megalocardia
meg ə lō kär′ dē ə

megal /o / cardi / a exists.

Megalocardia refers to heart muscle. When any muscle exercises, it gets larger. If the heart muscle has to overexercise,

Cardi/o/megal/y
cardiomegaly
kär dē ō meg′ ə lē
or
megal/o/cardi/a
megalocardia
meg ə lō kär′ dē ə

cardi /o / megal / y will probably occur. _megal /o / cardi /a_

Inadequate oxygen supply causes the heart muscle to beat more often. An inadequate amount of oxygen can lead to

megalocardia

megala cardia .

Prolonged, severe asthma can cut down the supply of oxygen to the body. This kind of asthma, if not checked, will cause

megalocardia

megalo cardia .

Megal/o/gastr/ia means large or enlarged stomach. The word root for stomach is _gastr_ .

gastr

megal/o means large, **gastr** is the word root for stomach, and **ia** is a noun ending. Form a noun that means large, or enlargement of the, stomach.

megal/o/gastr/ia
megalogastria
meg ə lō gas′ trē ə

megal /o / gastr /ia

Another word for enlargement of the stomach is gastr/o/megal/y. When the stomach is so large that it crowds other organs, a condition called

gastr/o/megal/y
gastromegaly
gas trō meg′ ə lē

megal/o/gastr/ia
megalogastria
meg ə lō gas′ trē ə

gastromegaly or
megalo gastria exists.

171

When the stomach is so large it crowds other organs, an undesirable condition known as _megalogastria, gastromegaly_ exists.

172

ia is a noun ending of condition. When megalogastria occurs, an undesirable _condition_ exists.

173

Mania is an English word that comes directly from the Greek word mania, which means madness. Many mental disorders are designated by compound words that end in this word, _mania_.

174

Man/ia is a noun of condition. The condition is "madness" or, more properly, mental disorder. The ending that tells you mania is a noun and shows a condition is _ia_.

175

Megal/o/man/ia is a symptom of a mental disorder in which the patient has delusions of grandeur. Patients who have greatly enlarged opinions of themselves suffer from _Megal / o / man / ia_.

megal/o/man/ia
megalomania
meg ə lō mā′ nē ə

176

People with megalomania are frequently found in mental hospitals. Many such hospitals have a patient who claims to be King Solomon. One of these patients's symptoms is _megalomania_.

177

Many people think Adolf Hitler suffered from delusions of grandeur or _megalomania_.

answer column	
enlargement of the heart heart	**178** Megal/o/cardi/a means ** <u>*enlarged heart*</u> _____. **cardi** is the word root for <u>*heart*</u> _____.
inflammation of the heart	**179** **cardi/o** is used in building words that refer to the heart. Card/itis means ** <u>*inflamed heart*</u> _____.
heart	**180** **logy** and **logist** are combining forms you will use as suffixes for convenience: logos —Greek for study log/y —noun, study of log/ist —noun, one who studies A cardi/o/logist is a specialist in the study of diseases of the <u>*heart*</u> _____.

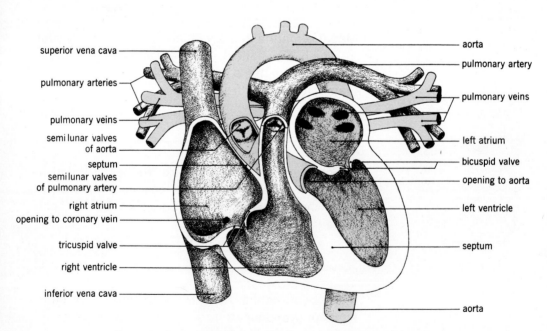

The heart (from Schifferes JJ, Peterson LJ: *Essentials of Healthier Living*, ed 4, New York, Wiley, 1972, p 282)

superior vena cava
pulmonary arteries
pulmonary veins
semilunar valves of aorta
septum
semilunar valves of pulmonary artery
right atrium
opening to coronary vein
tricuspid valve
right ventricle
inferior vena cava

aorta
pulmonary artery
pulmonary veins
left atrium
bicuspid valve
opening to aorta
left ventricle
septum
aorta

30

181

ic and **ac** are adjective suffixes. The following are adjectival forms of the words you have just learned:

    leukem/ic
    derm/ic
    man/ic
    gastr/ic
    cardi/ac

---

cardi/o/logist
cardiologist
kär dē ol′ ə jist

182

A/cardi/o/logist diagnoses heart disease (see Case Study page 33). The specialist who determines that a heart is deformed is a

cardi / o / logist .

---

cardiologist

183

A cardiologist discovers irregularities in the flow of the blood in the heart. The physician who catheterizes the heart is a _cardiologist_ .

---

cardiologist

184

A person who reads electr/o/cardi/o/grams (records of electrical impulses given off by the heart) is also a _cardiologist_ ,

---

a record of electrical
waves given off by the
heart
(or equivalent)

185

Give the meaning of electr/o/cardi/o/gram. (Gram/o is a combining form that means record.)
**

_____ .

---

electr/o/cardi/o/gram
electrocardiogram
e lek′ trō kär′ dē
o gram

186

Graph is a word root indicating an instrument used to make a recording or any pictorial device.
Electr/o/cardi/o/gram is the record produced. Electrocardiograph is the instrument used to record the picture, or _electro cardiagram_

---

electrocardiogram

187

The electr/o/cardi/o/gram is a record obtained by the process of electr/o/cardi/o/graph/y. A technician can learn electrocardiography, but it takes a cardiologist to read the
electocardiagram .

188

A physician can take a chart that looks like this,

ventricular fibrillation

complete heart block (atrial rate, 107; ventricular rate, 43)

and learn something about a person's heart. The physician is a _Cardiologist_ and is reading an _electrocardiogram_ .

189

algia is a suffix that means pain. Form a word that means heart pain. (Since algia is a suffix, you will use the word root rather than the combining form.)
_____ cardi / algia _____.

190

Gastr/algia means pain in the stomach. When a patient complains of pain in the heart, this symptom is known medically as
_____ cardialgia _____.

191

The suffix for pain is _algia_ .

192

Gastromegaly is one word for enlarged stomach. **gastr/o** is the combining form for _stomach_.

193

Gastr/ectomy means excision (removal) of all or part of the stomach. ectomy is a suffix meaning
_____ removal _____.

32

---

answer column	
	194 This is a free frame for those who are interested. Other may go on. 　ect/o　　combining form—outside 　 t om/e　cut 　　　y　noun ending 　ect om y　excision
gastr/ectomy gastrectomy gas trek′ tə mē	**195** A gastr/ectomy is a surgical procedure. When a stomach ulcer has perforated, a partial ___gastr / ectomy___ may be indicated.
gastrectomy	**196** Cancer of the stomach may be treated by a ___gastrectomy___ .
gastr/itis gastritis gas trī′ tis	**197** Form a word that means inflammation of the stomach. ___gastr / itis___

33

answer column	

Two words that mean enlargement of the stomach are _megal/o/gastr/ia_ and _gastr/o/megal/y_.

199

duoden/o is used in words that refer to the first part of the small intestine, the duoden/um. To build words about the duodenum, use

duoden/o .

An outline of terms and illustration showing the digestive system follows Frame 710.

duoden/o

200

The duoden/um is the part of the small intestine that connects with the stomach. Duoden/o is a word root-combining form that refers to the

duoden / um .

duoden/um
dōō ō dē nəm,
dōō od′ ə nəm

201

Gastr/o/duoden/ostomy means formation of a new opening between the stomach and duodenum. **ostomy** is a combining form you can use as a suffix to mean **forming an opening.** Gastr/o/duoden/ostomy means **_____

_____ .

forming an opening
between the stomach
and duodenum

202

Here's another free frame for those interested in ostomy.

ost/i	mouth—opening
tom/e	cut
y	noun ending
make a **mouth**	(opening) by cutting

203

Gastr/o/duoden/ostomy means forming an opening between the stomach and duodenum. A surgeon who removes the natural connection between the duodenum and stomach, and then forms a new connection, is doing a

gastr /o/ duoden /ostomy

gastr/o/duoden/ostomy
gastroduodenostomy
gas′ trō dōō ō də nos′
tə mē

34

204

A gastroduodenostomy is a surgical procedure. When the pyloric sphincter, a valve that controls the amount of food going from the stomach to the duodenum, no longer functions, a _gastro duodenostomy_ may be done.

205

When a portion of the first part of the small intestine is removed because of cancer, a new opening is formed by performing a

_____.

206

o/tom/y is a combining form you may use as a suffix because it connects directly to a word root. A duo/den/otomy is an incision into the _duodenum_.

207

If a duo/den/otomy is an incision into the duodenum, the part meaning **incision** is _otomy_.

208

otomy means incision into. An incision into the duodenum is a _duoden/otomy_.

209

If a growth has to be removed from the inner wall of the duodenum, a _duodenotomy_ is done.

210

A surgeon who incises the duodenum is performing a _duodenotomy_.

itis
duoden/itis
duodenitis
doo̅ o̅ də ni̅′ tis,
doo̅ od ə ni̅′ tis

211

The suffix for inflammation is _itis_. The word for inflammation of the duodenum is _duoden/ itis_.

212

itis indicates a general symptomatic term. When physicians are listing symptoms about the duodenum and they want to say it is inflamed, they use the word _duodenitis_.

duodenitis

213

Duoden/al is an adjective. **al** is an adjectival ending meaning pertaining to (whatever the adjective modifies). One adjectival ending is _al_.

al

214

duoden/al duodenal
dōō ō dē′ nəl,
doo od′ ə nəl
ulcer
lesion

In **duoden/al ulcer** and **duoden/al lesion,** the adjective is _duoden/_ and the nouns modified are _ulcer_ and _lesion_.

(See "Case Study: Endoscopy Report" on opposite page.)

215

In the sentence, "Duodenal carcinoma was present," the adjective meaning pertaining to the duodenum is _duodenal_.

duodenal

216

The adjectival form of duoden/o is _duodenal_.

duodenal

217

duoden/ostomy
duodenostomy
dōō ō də nos′ tə mē

ostomy means making a new opening. The word to form a new opening into the duodenum is _duoden / ostomy_.

218

A duodenostomy **can** be formed in more than one manner. If it is formed with the stomach, it is called a _gastroduodenostomy_.

gastroduodenostomy

219

The suffix for forming a new opening is _ostomy_.

ostomy

CASE STUDY: ENDOSCOPY REPORT

DIAGNOSIS: Gastrointestinal hemorrhage, presumably a duodenal ulcer.

SUMMARY: This patient is a 89-year-old female admitted through the hospital emergency room because of vomiting coffee ground material and passing melanic stools. The naso-gastric tube inserted in this patient showed bright red blood. Subsequently, the patient became hypotensive and two units of packed red cells were given. The patient then became stable, with a blood pressure of 120/80. She was lavaged with iced isotonic saline and an endoscopy was performed.

ENDOSCOPY: *Premedication:* Catacaine locally. A Fiberscope Olympus Q was easily passed into the esophagus. Numerous amounts of clots were noted. The scope was introduced into the stomach, which showed increased amounts of bright red blood in the fundus. No mucosal lesions could be seen; however, half of the stomach was full of blood. The scope was then passed into the duodenal bulb, where clots were also noted. This patient could have a duodenal ulcer, but because of the amount of blood, it is difficult to delineate an ulcer crater. A great clot is located on the anterior wall. As the scope is withdrawn, the antrum of the stomach can be seen with no lesion noted. It was difficult to clean up all the blood clots, and because of the status of the patient, the examination was stopped. However, the patient tolerated the procedure very well and did not vomit or aspirate.

Use the material in the following chart to work the next seven frames.

WORDS ARE FORMED BY
I. Word root + suffix
a. dermat/itis
b. cyan/osis
c. duoden/al
II. Combining form + word root + suffix
(this can be a word itself)
a. acr/o/cyan/osis
b. leuk/o/cyte
III. Any number of combining forms + word root + suffix
a. leuk/o/cyt/o/pen/ia
b. electr/o/cardi/o/graph/y

answer column	
word root	**220**
	In I(a) dermat is the * word root ;
suffix	itis is the ___suffix___ .
word root	**221**
suffix	In I(b) cyan is the * word root ;
	osis is the ___suffix___ .

37

222

duoden	In I(c) the word root is _____ ;
al	the suffix is _____ .

223

combining form	In II(a) acr/o is the *_____ ;
word root	cyan is the *_____ ;
suffix	osis is the _____ .

224

combining form	In II(b) leuk/o is the *_____ ;
word root	cyt is the *_____ ;
suffix	e is the _____ .

225

combining form	In III(a) leuk/o is a *_____ ;
combining form	cyt/o is a *_____ ;
word root	pen is a *_____ ;
suffix	ia is a _____ .

Work Review Sheets 1 and 2 (in Appendix A).

✗ study this too

226

electr/o	In III(b) the first combining form is ____electr / o__ ;
cardi/o	the second combining form is ____cardi / o__ ;
graph	the word root is __graph__ ;
y	the suffix that makes it a noun is __y__ .

227

You can form words without even knowing the meaning in the next four frames. Use what is needed from encephal/o + itis to form a word:

encephal/itis   __encephal / o itis__

38

228

Use what is needed from   encephal/o
malac/o
ia

encephal/o/malac/ia   *encephal /o /malac / /a*

---

encephal/o/mening/
itis

229

Use what is needed from   encephal/o
mening/o
itis

encephal /o / mening / it's

230

Use what is needed from   encephal/o
myel/o
path/o
y

encephal/o/myel/o/
path/y   *encephal / o / myel /o / pATh / y*

231

A prefix goes before a word to change its meaning. In the words hyper/trophy, hyper/emia, and hyper/emesis, hyper changes the meaning of trophy, emia, and emesis. **hyper** is a ___*prefix*___.

prefix

232

hyper is a prefix that means above or more than normal. To say that a person was overly critical, you would use the word

hyper   *hyper*/   critic   /   al___.

233

hypo is a prefix that is just the opposite of **hyper.** The prefix for under or less than normal is

hypo   *hypo*___.

---

hypo/trophy
hypotrophy
hī pot′ rə fē

234

The word root-combining form for growth or development is **troph/o.** Hypo/trophy means progressive degeneration. When an organ or tissue that has developed properly wastes away or decreases in size, it is undergoing ___*hypo*___ / *trophy*.

39

answer column

235

Hypotrophy occurs in many tissues. When muscles are not nourished or exercised, they undergo _hypotrophy_.

hypotrophy

236

As a result of weight lifting, body builder's muscles overdevelop, or _hypertrophy_.

hyper/troph/y

237

derm/o refers to _skin_. derm/ic makes the word an adjective. Hypo/derm/ic is an adjective that means under the _skin_.

skin

skin

238

In hypo/derm/ic, **ic** as a suffix forms a(n) _adj_ (adjective/noun). A needle that is inserted under the skin is a _hypo/derm/ic_ needle.

adjective
hypo/derm/ic
hypodermic
hī pō dûr′ mik

239

A hypodermic needle is short because it goes just under the skin into the subcutaneous layer. An injection that can be given superficially is administered with a _hypodermic_ needle. (See illustration of injections following frame _1253_.

hypodermic

240

In hypodermic, the prefix is _hypo_ and means _under_; the suffix is _ic_ and forms an _adjective_ (part of speech).

hypo
under
ic
adjective

241

Hyper/thyroid/ism means overactivity of the thyroid gland. The prefix that means the thyroid gland is secreting more than normal is _hyper_.

hyper

242

Emesis is a word that means vomiting. A word that means excessive vomiting is _hyper/emesis_.

hyper/emesis
hyperemesis
hī pər em′ ə sis

40

answer column	

243

Hyperemesis gravidarum is a complication of pregnancy that can require hospitalization. The part of the disorder that tells you excessive vomiting occurs is _____hyper emesis_____.

hyperemesis

244

Gallbladder attacks can cause excessive vomiting. This, too, is called

_____hyperemesis_____.

hyperemesis

245

Hyper/trophy means overdevelopment. Troph/o comes from the Greek word for nourishment. See the connection between nourishment and development. Overdevelopment is called

_____hyper_____ / _____trophy_____.

hyper/trophy
hypertrophy
hī pûr′ trə fē

246

Many organs can hypertrophy. If the heart overdevelops, the condition is _____hypertrophy_____ of the heart.

hypertrophy

247

Muscles also can overdevelop or

_____hypertrophy_____.

hypertrophy

248

aden/o is used in words that refer to glands. The word root is _____aden_____. The combining form is _____aden_____ / _____o_____.

aden

aden/o

249

Build a word that means inflammation of a gland (word root + suffix rule)

_____aden_____ / _____itis_____

(See "Operative Report" following frame ___123___)

aden/itis
adenitis
ad ə ni′ tis

250

Aden/ectomy means excision or removal of a gland. The part that means excision is

_____adenectomy_____.

ectomy

41

answer column

answer column	
aden aden/ectomy adenectomy ad ə nek′ tə mē	The part that means gland is _aden_. The word for removal of a gland is _aden / ectomy_.

251

An adenectomy is a surgical procedure. If a gland is tumorous, part or all of it may be excised. This operation is an _adenectomy_.

adenectomy

252

A tumor is an abnormal growth of cells also referred to as a neoplasm. **oma** is the suffix for tumor. Form a word that means tumor of a gland.

adenoma

aden/oma

253

Sometimes the thyroid gland develops an adenoma. In this case, a patient's history might read, " . . . hyperthyroidism noted—due to presence of a thyroid _aden oma_ ."

adenoma

254

When a thyroid _adenoma_ (tumor of a gland) is found, a partial _adenectomy_ (excision of gland) is performed.

adenoma
adenectomy or
(thyroidectomy)

255

path/o is the combining form for disease. Aden/o/path/y means any disease of a gland. In this word you have a combining form + a* _word root_ _____ + a suffix to form the word _aden /o /path /y_ .

word root
aden/o/path/y
adenopathy
ad ə nop′ ə thē

256

Adenopathy means glandular disease in general. When the diagnosis is made of a diseased gland, but the disease is not specifically known or stated, the word used is _adenopathy_ .

adenopathy

42

answer column	

adenopathy

adenoma

adenectomy

257

An ___adenopathy___ (glandular disease) could be diagnosed as an ___adenoma___ (glandular tumor). If so, the surgeon may want to have an ___adenectomy___ (excision of a gland) performed.

---

adenitis

adenectomy

258

When a gland is found to have a mild ___adenitis___ (inflammation), no ___adenectomy___ (surgery) is indicated.

---

tumor

fat

259

An adenoma is a glandular tumor. **oma** is the suffix for ___tumor___. A lip/oma is a tumor containing fat. Lip/o is the word root–combining form for ___fat___.

---

lip/oma

līp ō′ mə

260

A lip/oma is usually benign (noncancerous). A fatty tumor is called a ___lip / o / ma___.

---

cancerous tumor or malignant tumor

261

carcin/o is the word root–combining form for cancer. A carcin/oma is a

** ___cancerous tumor___ .

---

carcinoma

262

A carcinoma may occur in almost any part of the body. A stomach cancer is called gastric ___carcinoma___ .

---

carcinoma

kär sin ō′ mə

263

Carcinoma may metastasize (spread to other parts of the body) through the bloodstream. The intestine has a rich blood supply. For this reason, intestinal ___carcinoma___ is extremely dangerous.

---

carcinoma

264

Carcinoma may be confined to the site of its origin. In this case, it is called ___carcinoma___ in situ.

TUMOR TERMINOLOGY

COMBINING FORM	MEANING	TERM
aden/o	gland	adenoma
lip/o	fat	lipoma
melan/o	black	melanoma
granul/o	granular tissue	granuloma
neur/o	nerve	neuroma
my/o	muscle	myoma
oste/o	bone	osteoma
lymph/o	lymph tissue	lymphoma
carcin/o	cancer	carcinoma
sarc/o	malignant connective tissue	sarcoma
papill/o	small elevation of tissue	papilloma

aden/o/carcinoma
adenocarcinoma
ad′ ē nō kär sin ō′ ma

265
Form a word that means cancer of glandular tissue.
aden /o / carcinom/a

lip/o

lip/oid
lipoid
lip′ oid

266
The combining form for fat is _lip / o_.
oid is a suffix that means like or resembling. Build a word which means fatlike or resembling fat.
lip / oid

fat
lipoid

267
The word lipoid is used in chemistry or pathology. It describes a substance that looks like fat, dissolves like fat, but is not _fat_. A word that means resembling fat is _lipoid_.

lipoid

268
In proper amounts cholesterol is essential to health, but too much may cause arteriosclerosis. Cholesterol is an alcohol that resembles fat; therefore, it is a _lipoid_.

resembling
muc
muc/o

269
Muc/oid means resembling mucus. **oid** is a suffix meaning _resembling_. The word root for mucus is _muc_, and its combining form is _muc/ o_.

44

270

Mucoid is an adjective that means resembling or like mucus. There is a substance in connective tissue that resembles mucus. This is a

muc / _oid_ substance.

271

There is a protein in the body that resembles mucus. This protein is said to be _mucoid_ in nature.

mucoid

272

Anything that resembles mucus is called

mucoid.

mucoid

273

Muc/us is a secretion of the muc/ous membrane. **us** is a noun suffix. **ous** is an adjectival suffix. The muc/ous membrane secretes _muc_ / _us_.

muc/us
mucus
myoo′ kəs

274

Mucus is secreted by cells in the nose. It traps dust and bacteria from the air. One of the body's protective devices is _mucus_.

mucus

275

The mucous membrane secretes _mucus_.
The tissue that secretes mucus is the

muc / _ous_ membrane or muc/osa.

mucus
muc/ous
mucous
myoo′ kəs

276

The noun (the secretion) built from muc/o is _mucus_. The adjective (pertaining to) built from muc/o is _mucous_.

mucus
mucous

277

The mucous membrane or mucosa is found lining the body openings. This protective, mucous membrane can also be called the _muc_ / _osa_:

muc/osa

278

The mucosa secretes _mucus_. Anything that resembles mucus is _mucoid_. Mucoid

mucus
mucoid

mucosa or
mucous membrane

substances are not mucus; therefore, they are not secreted by the

** _mucosa_ .

279

At this stage of word building, students sometimes find that they have one big pain in the head. The word for pain in the head is cephal/algia. The word root for head is _cephal_ .

cephal

280

algia

One suffix for pain is _algia_ .

281

cephal/algia
cephalalgia
sef ə lal′ jē ə

If you are suffering from cephalalgia, persevere, for later this gets to be fun. Any pain in the head may be called

cephal / _algia_ .

282

cephalalgia

The word root–combining form for head is cephal/o. The word for pain in the head is

cephalalgia .

283

cephal/o/dyn/ia
cephalodynia
sef ə lō din′ ē ə

cephal/algia

Another word for pain in the head is cephal/o/dyn/ia. This word shows the combining form before the word root + a suffix. If this seems a headache, relax. Either word,

cephal / _o_ / _dyn_ / _ia_

or _cephal_ / _algia_ will do for headache.

284

dyn/ia

algia

algia and **dyn/ia** are usually interchangeable. The combining form requires _dyn/ia_ , while a word root takes the suffix _algia_ .

285

cephal/o/dyn/ic
cephalodynic
sef ə lō din′ ik

dynia can take the adjectival form dyn/ic. An adjective that means pertaining to head pain is

cephal / _o_ / _dyn_ / _ic_ .

46

answer column

286

To say medically that headache discomfort exists, use the adjective

cephal/o/dyn/ic *(handwritten)*

for headache.

cephal/o/dyn/ic

287

Two nouns for head pain are

cephalalgia *(handwritten)* and

cephalodynia *(handwritten)* .

The adjective used for head pain is

cephalodynic *(handwritten)* .

cephalalgia
cephalodynia

cephalodynic

288

Cephal/ic means pertaining to or toward the head. Cephal/ic is a(n) adjective *(handwritten)*
(noun/adjective). This is evident because cephalic ends in ic *(handwritten)* .

adjective

ic

289

Cephalic is an adjective. A case history reporting head cuts due to an accident might read,
" cephal/ic *(handwritten)* lacerations present."

cephal/ic
cephalic
sə fal′ ik

290

In the phrase, "lack of cephalic orientation," the adjective is cephalic *(handwritten)* .

cephalic

291

Another phrase might be, " cephalic *(handwritten)*
tumors noted."

cephalic

292

Inside the head **en**closed in bone, is the brain. **encephal/o** is used in words pertaining to the brain. Build a word meaning inflammation of the brain.

encepha/litis *(handwritten)*

encephal/itis
encephalitis
en sef ə lī′ tis

293

The suffix for tumor is oma *(handwritten)* . Use what is necessary from encephal/o to build a word for brain tumor. encephal/oma *(handwritten)*

oma
encephal/oma
encephaloma
en sef ə lō′ mə

47

294

The Greek word for hernia is kele; the suffix is cele. Encephal/o/cele is a word meaning herniation of _____*brain*_____ tissue.

295

An encephalocele occurs when some brain tissue protrudes through a cranial fissure (see illustration page 51). The word for herniation of brain tissue is ___*encephal* / *o* / *cele*___.

encephal/o/cele
encephalocele
en sef′ ə lō sēl

296

Any hernia is a projection of a part from its natural cavity. Herniation is indicated by **cele.** A projection of brain tissue from its natural cavity is an ___*encephal* / *o* / *cele*___.

297

Brain herniation is sometimes a symptom of hydro-cephaly. This symptom, in medical language, is called an ___*encephalocele*___.

298

The noun for protrusion of brain tissue through a cranial fissure is ___*encephalocele*___.

299

Malac/ia is a word meaning softening of a tissue. Encephal/o/malac/ia means ** ___*brain tissue softening*___.

300

malac/o is the combining form. The word root is ___*malac*___.

301

Encephal/o/malac/ia ends in **ia. ia** is a suffix that forms a noun. A noun meaning softening of brain tissue is ___*encephal* / *o* / *malac* / *ia*___.

encephal/o/malac/ia
encephalomalacia
en sef ə lō mə lā′ shə

302

An accident causing brain injury could result in the softening of some brain tissue, or

encephalomalacia *encephalomalacia*.

303

Some brain diseases can also cause softening and produce the symptom,

encephalomalacia *encephalomalacia*.

304

otomy is used as a suffix for making an incision or temporary opening. An incision into the brain is an

encephal/o/tomy
encephalotomy
en sef ə lot′ ō mē *encephal/o/tomy*.

305

Using what is necessary from malac/o with the suffix otomy, form a word that means incision of soft areas.

malac/otomy
malacotomy
mal ə kot′ ə mē *malac/otomy*

coronal suture

parietal bone

frontal bone

superciliary arch
sphenoid bone

temporal bone

occipital bone

nasal bone
lacrimal bone
zygomatic process

external
occipital
protuberance

zygomatic arch
zygoma

mastoid process

maxilla

mental foramen
mandible

Lateral view of cranium

surgical repair of the skull or cranium	**306** **crani/o** is used in words referring to the crani/um or skull. Crani/o/plast/y means ** _____ _____.
crani/o/malac/ia craniomalacia krā nē ō mə lā′ shə	**307** The word for softening of the bones of the skull is _____ / _____ / _____ / _____.
crani/ectomy craniectomy krā nē ek′ tə mē	**308** The word meaning **excision** of part of the cranium is _crani_ / _ectomy_.
crani/otomy craniotomy krā nē ot′ ə mē	**309** The word for **incision** into the skull is _crani_ / _otomy_.
crani/o/meter craniometer krā nē om′ ə tər	**310** An instrument to measure the cranium is the _crani_ / _o_ / _meter_.
cranial cranial	**311** There are cranial bones. There are also _cranial_ nerves. There are grooves and furrows called _cranial_ fissures.
adjectival	**312** Crani/al is the _adjectival_ (noun/adjectival) form of crani/o.
cerebr/um cerebrum ser′ ə brəm sə rē′ brəm	**313** Crani/o/cerebr/al refers to the skull and the cerebr/um. The cerebr/um is a part of the brain. Cerebr/o is used to build words about the _cerebrum_.
cerebrum	**314** The cerebrum is the part of the brain in which thought occurs. Humans can think. Generally speaking, other animals cannot. Humans have a better-developed _cerebrum_ than other animals.

50

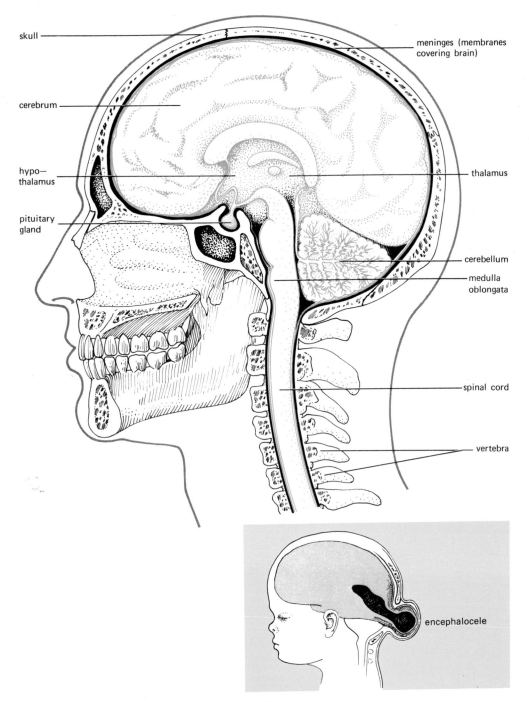

skull

meninges (membranes covering brain)

cerebrum

hypo—thalamus

thalamus

pituitary gland

cerebellum

medulla oblongata

spinal cord

vertebra

encephalocele

The Brain

51

answer column	
	315
cerebrum	Feeling is interpreted in the cerebrum. Motor impulses also arise in the _cerebrum_ .
	316
cerebrum	Thinking, feeling, and movement are controlled by the gray matter of the _cerebrum_ . (Were you ever told to use your "gray matter"? This is why.)
cerebr/al cerebral ser′ ə brəl, sə rē′ brəl	**317** The adjectival form of cerebrum is _cerebr/al_ .
cerebral	**318** There is a cerebral reflex. There are cerebral fissures. You have probably heard of _cerebral_ hemorrhage.
inflammation of the cerebrum	**319** Cerebr/itis means ** _inflamed cerebrum_ .
cerebral tumor or any mass in the brain	**320** A cerebr/oma is a ** _tumor of the brain_ .
cerebr/otomy cerebrotomy ser ə brot′ ə mē	**321** An incision into the cerebrum to remove an abscess is a _cerebr /otomy_ .
cerebr/o/spin/al cerebrospinal ser ə brō spī′ nəl	**322** Cerebr/o/spin/al refers to the brain and spinal cord. There is fluid that bathes the cerebrum and spinal cord. It is _cerebr/o / spin /al_ fluid.
cerebrospinal	**323** A cerebr/o/spin/al puncture is sometimes done to remove _cerebro spinal_ fluid.

52

answer column	
cerebrospinal	**324** There is even a disease called _cerebrospinal_ meningitis.
mening/es· meninges me nin′ jēz	**325** The meninges is a three-layered membrane that covers the brain and spinal cord. These three layers are the pia mater, arachnoid, and dura mater. The protective covering of the brain and spinal cord is the _meninges_.
mening/o/cele meningocele me nin′ gō sēl	**326** A herniation of the meninges is a _mening / o / cele_.
meninges	**327** A meningocele is a herniation of the _meninges_.
meninges	**328** Mening/o/malac/ia means softening of the _meninges_.
mening/itis meningitis men in jī′ tis	**329** Mening/itis can occur as cerebr/al meningitis, as spin/al mening/itis, or as cerebr/o/spin/al _mening/itis_.
meningitis	**330** There are many kinds of meningitis. The tubercle bacillus can cause tuberculous meningitis. Mening/o/cocc/i are bacteria that cause epidemic. _meningitis_.

Work Review Sheets 3 and 4.

oste/o	**331** Osteopathy means disease of the bones. From this word form the word root-combining form for bone. _oste / o_

332

A word meaning inflammation of bones is

_____oste /itis_____ .

333

Oste/o/malac/ia means softening of the bones. To say that bones have lost a detectable amount of their hardness, use the noun

_____Oste / o / malac / ia .

oste/o/malac/ia
osteomalacia
os tē ō mə lā′/ shə

334

One cause of oste/o/malac/ia is the removal of calcium from the bones. When calcium is removed from the bones and they lose some of their hardness, a disorder called

_____Oste / o / malac/ i a_____

results.

335

A disorder of the parathyroid gland can cause calcium to be withdrawn from the bones. When this occurs,

_____oste omalacia_____ ,

results.

336

When there is not enough calcium in the diet, this same disorder, ____osteomalacia____, can occur.

337

Form a word that means disease of bone.

_____oste / o / path / y_____

338

A hard outgrowth on a bone may be a bone tumor or ____oste/ oma____ .

339

path/o means disease. Oste/o/arthr/o/path/y is a noun that means any disease involving bones and joints. **arthr/o** is used in words to mean _____joint_____ .

answer column	
	340
	Oste/o/arthr/o/path/y is a compound noun. Analyze it:
oste/o	_oste / o_ bone (combining form)
arthr/o	_arthr / o_ joint (combining form)
path	_path_ disease (word root)
y	_y_ noun (suffix)
oste/o/arthr/o/path/y	Now put it together:
osteoarthropathy	_oste / o / arthr / o / path / y_
os tē ō är throp′ ə thē	
	341
any disease of the	Cerebr/o/path/y means ** _disease of_
cerebrum; or disease	_the cerebrum_ .
of the cerebrum	
	342
	An instrument used to look at something is a scope.
arthr/o/scope	An instrument used to look into a joint is an
arthroscope	_arthr / o / scope_ .
är′ thrō skōp	
	343
	The name of the procedure for examining the joints
arthr/o/scop/y	by looking with an arthroscope is called
arthroscopy	_arthroscopy_ .
är thro′ skō pē	
	344
	Arthr/o/plast/y means surgical repair of a joint.
	Plast/y means
surgical repair	* _surgical repair_ .
	345
	Think of a plast/ic surgeon building a new nose
	or doing a face-lifting. These are surgical repairs.
	Plast/o means
surgical repair	* _surgical repair_ .
	346
	Arthr/o/plast/y may take many forms. When a joint
	has lost its ability to move, movement can some-
	times be restored by an
arthr/o/plast/y	_arthr / o / plast / y_ .

55

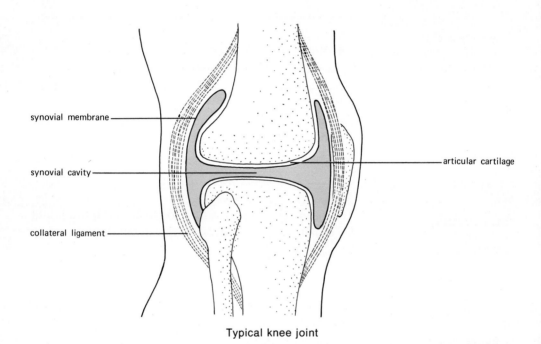

Typical knee joint

synovial membrane

synovial cavity

collateral ligament

articular cartilage

347
Arthroplasty is a noun. If a child is born without a joint, sometimes one can be formed by a surgical procedure called

arthroplasty

arthroplasty .

---

arthr/itis
arthritis
är thrī′ tis

348
Form a word that means inflammation of a joint.

arthr / itis

---

arthr/otomy
arthrotomy
är throt′ ə mē

349
You're getting to be pretty good at this, aren't you? Form a word that means incision of a joint.

arthr / otomy

---

ten/o/plast/y
ten′ ō plas tē
ten/o/dyn/ia
ten ō din′ ē ə

350
Ten/o means tendons. Build a word meaning:

repair of tendons _ten / o / plast / y_ ;

pain in tendons _ten / o / dyn / ia_ .

56

answer column	

burs/itis
bûr sī′ tis

burs/ectomy
bûr sek′ tə mē

351

A bursa is a small serous sac between a tendon and a bone. Burs/o refers to the bursae of the body. Build a word meaning:

inflammation of a bursa _burs/itis_ ;

excision of a bursa _burs/ectomy_ .

---

chondr/o

352

The word oste/o/chondr/itis means inflammation of bone and cartilage. The word root–combining form for cartilage is _chondr/o_ .

---

cartilage

353

Cartilage is a tough, elastic connective tissue found in the ear, nose tip, and rib ends. The lining of joints also contains _cartilage_ .

---

chondr/algia
chondr/o/dyn/ia

You pronounce.

354

Form a word meaning pain in or around cartilage.

chondr/algia

(word root + suffix) or

condr/o/dyn/ia

(combining form for cartilage).

---

ten/o/plast/y
ten′ ō plas tē

ten/o/dyn/ia
ten ō din′ ē ə

355

Ten/o means tendons. Build a word meaning:

repair of tendons _ten/o/plast/y_ ;

pain in tendons _ten/o/dyn/ia_ .

---

excision of cartilage

356

Chondr/ectomy means

** _excision of cartilage_ .

---

ribs

357

Chondr/o/cost/al means pertaining to rib cartilage. **cost/o** is used in words about the _rib_ .

---

cost/ectomy
costectomy
kos tek′ tə mē

358

Form a word that means excision of a rib or ribs.

cost/ectomy

359

Chondr/o/cost/al is an adjective. This is evident because **al** is the ending for an

_____*adjective*_____.

360

Chondrocost/al means pertaining to the ribs and cartilage. **al** forms an adjective that means

* _____*pertaing to*_____.

361

Analyze chondr/o/cost/al:

_____*Chondr/o*_____ cartilage

_____*cost*_____ rib

_____*al*_____ suffix

Now put them together:

_____*chondr/o/cost/al*_____.

This means * _____*pertaing to rib cartilage*_____
_____.

362

Form a word that means pertaining to the ribs.

_____*cost/al*_____

363

Inter/cost/al means between the ribs. The prefix

for between is _____*Inter*_____.

364

inter/chondr/al
interchondral
in tər kon′ drəl

Form a word that means between cartilages.

_____*Inter / chondr / al*_____

(adjective)

365

Inter/cost/al means between the ribs. **inter** is the

prefix that means _____*between*_____.

366

Inter/cost/al may refer to the muscles between the ribs. These muscles that move the ribs when breath-

inter/cost/al
intercostal
in tər kos′ təl

ing are the

_____*inter / cost / al*_____ muscles.

58

answer column

intercostal

dent

between the teeth

inter/dent/al
interdental
in tər den' təl

interdental

dent/al
dental
den' təl

dent/algia
dentalgia
den tal' jē ə

dent/oid
dentoid
den' toid

teeth
teeth

367

One set of intercostal muscles enlarges the rib cage when one is breathing in. When one exhales, the rib cage is made smaller by another set of _intercostal_ muscles.

368

Inter/dent/al means between the teeth. The word root for tooth is _dent_.

369

An inter/dent/al cavity occurs
** _between the teeth_.

370

Inter/dent/al is an adjective so it must modify a noun. In "interdental spaces" the adjective is
inter / dent / al.

371

In "interdental cavity" the adjective is
interdental.

372

Form an adjective that means pertaining to the teeth. _dent/al_

373

Pain in the teeth, or a toothache, is called
dent/algia.

374

oid is the suffix that means like or resembling. Form a word that means tooth-shaped or resembling a tooth. _dent/oid_

375

A dent/ist takes care of _teeth_.
A dent/ifrice is used for cleaning _teeth_.

59

376

lumb/o builds words about the loin. Lumb/ar is the adjectiv/al form. An **adjective** meaning pertaining to the loin is ___*lumb/ar*___.

377

There are five lumb/ar vertebrae. Low back (loin) pain is called ___*lumbar*___ pain.

378

There is also a reflex called the ___*lumbar*___ reflex.

379

Thorac/o/lumb/ar is a(n) ___*adj.*___ (noun/adjective) meaning ** ___*pertaining to the chest + loin*___.

adjective
pertaining to the chest
  and loin or something
  near this

380

supra is a prefix that means on, higher in position, outside, or further.

381

Supra/lumb/ar means above the lumbar region. A prefix that means above is ___*supra*___.

382

Supra/lumb/ar means ** ___*above the loin*___.

383

Supra/cost/al means
** ___*above the ribs*___.

384

Supra/crani/al refers to the surface of the head ** ___*on top of*___ the skull.

385

Supra/pub/ic means above the pubis. Pub/o is used in words about the ___*pubis*___.

60

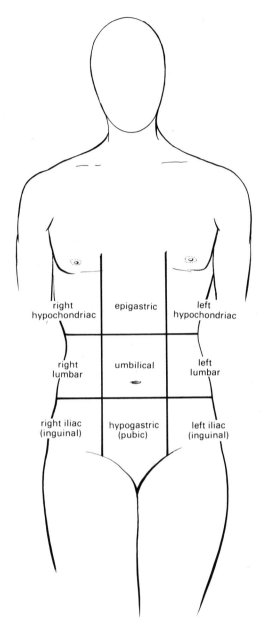

Regions of the abdomen

supra/pub/ic
suprapubic
soo prə pyoo′ bik

386

The suprapubic region is above the arch of the pub/is. When the bladder is incised above the pubis, an incision is made in the

_____ supra / bub / ic _____ region.

61

387

"The incision is made in the suprapubic region." From this sentence pick out

suprapubic
incision
region

the adjective: _Supra pubic_ ;

two nouns: _inscision_ ,

region .

388

suprapubic

There is also a reflex called the _supra pubic_ reflex.

389

anything close to
  incision of bladder from
  the suprapubic region

Try to figure out what surgery is done in a **supra/ pubic cyst/otomy** ** _____

_____ .

390

noun

The pub/is is a bone of the pelvis. Pub/is is a _noun_ (noun/adjective).

391

pubis
pubic

From pub/o form   a noun: _pubis_ ;

an adjective: _pubic_ .

(See illustration following frame _1401_ .

392

pubis

The pub/ic bone is also called the _pubis_ .

393

pelv/is
pelvis
pel' vis

The pelv/is is formed by the pelv/ic bones. Pelv/i refers to the _pelv/is_ (noun).

394

pelv/i/metr/y
pelvimetry
pel vim' ə tre

Pelv/i/metr/y is done during pregnancy to find the measurements of the pelvis. To find a woman's pelvic size, the physician does

pelv/i/metr/y .

395

pelvimetry

Look up pelvimetry or pelvis in your dictionary. Taking pelvic measurements is called

pelvimetry .

answer column

396

A physician may determine whether or not a woman will have trouble during labor by doing

pelvimetry

pelvimetry .

397

Look in the dictionary for a word that names the device used for pelvimetry. It is a

pelv/i/meter
pelvimeter
pel vim' ə tər

pelvimeter .

398

The pelvimeter measures different diameters. Pelvimetry is done by reading a scale of numbers on

pelvimeter

the _pelvimeter_ .

399

pelvimeter

To measure the pelvis, the _pelvimeter_ is used.

400

A meter is an instrument to measure.

instrument

A speed/o/meter is an _instrument_ to measure speed.

instrument

A pelv/i/meter is an _instrument_ to measure the pelvis.

401

measures

A cyt/o/meter _measures_ cells.

measures
thorac/o/meter
thôr ə kom' ə tər
cardi/o/meter
kär dē om' ə tər

A cephal/o/meter _measures_ the skull.

A _thora /o / meter_ measures the chest.

A _cardi /o / meter_ measures the heart.

402

supra/pelv/ic
suprapelvic
soo prə pel' vik

The adjective meaning **above** the pelvis is

supra / pelv / ic .

403

Ab/norm/al is a word that means deviating (turning away) from what is normal. **ab** is a

pre

pre fix that means **from.**

63

404

Ab/normal is used in ordinary English. If abnormal is in your usable vocabulary, skip this frame. If you have **never** used the word abnormal, write it five times.

ab/normal

abnormal

ab nôr′ məl

_____   _____

_____   _____

_____

405

ab is a prefix that means from or away from. Ab-normal means * <u>away from normal</u> normal.

away from

406

ab is a prefix that means

from or away from

* <u>away from</u> .

407

Ab/errant uses the prefix ab before the English word for wandering. Ab/errant means ** <u>wandering from</u> .

wandering from (the normal course of events)

408

Ab/errant is used in medicine to describe a structure that wanders from the normal. When some nerve fibers follow an unusual route, they form an <u>ab / errant</u> nerve.

ab/errant

aberrant

ab er′ ənt

409

Aberrant nerves wander from the normal nerve track. Blood vessels that follow a path of their own are <u>aberrant</u> vessels.

aberrant

410

Lymph vessels may be found in unexpected areas of the body. They follow an <u>aberrant</u> course.

aberrant

411

Ab/duct/ion means movement away from a midline. When the arm is raised away from the side of the body <u>ab / duct / ion</u> has occurred.

ab/duct/ion

64

answer column

abduction
ab duk shun

abducted

ad/duction
adduction
ə duk′ shən

ad/diction
addiction
ə dik′ shən

addiction

addict

ad/hesion
adhesion
ad hē′ zhən

adhesions

adhesions

412
Abduction can occur from any midline. When the fingers of the hand are spread apart, _abduction_ has occurred in four fingers.

413
A child who has been kidnapped and taken away from home has been ___abducted___ (past tense verb).

414
ad is a prefix meaning toward. Movement toward a midline is ___ad/ duction___.

415
Addiction means being drawn toward some habit. The person who takes drugs habitually suffers from drug ___ad/ diction___.

416
Addiction implies habit. Alcoholism is ___addiction___ to alcohol.

417
A person addicted to drugs is a drug addict. A person addicted to cocaine is a cocaine ___addict___.

418
An ad/hesion is formed when two normally separate tissues join together. They adhere to each other. Adhering to another part forms an ___ad/ hesion___.

419
Some years ago, adhesions occurred frequently following surgery. Patients did not walk soon enough, so tissues healed together. Following an appendectomy, ___adhesions___ were common.

420
Now patients walk on the day after an appendectomy. This has practically eliminated ___adhesions___.

421
Patients walk within a day after most abdominal surgery. This has nearly eliminated ___adhesions___.

adhesions

422
abdomin/o is used to form words about the abdomen. When you see abdomin/o any place in a word, you think about the ___abdomen___.

abdomen
ab′ də mən, ab dō′ mən

423
Abdomin/al is an adjective that means ** ___
___pertaining to the abdomen___.

pertaining to the
    abdomen

424
Look up the word **paracentesis** in your dictionary. Write the definition here.
___a procedure in which fluid is___
___drawn from the body___

The insertion of a needle
    into a body cavity
    for the purpose of
    aspirating fluid

425
Abdomin/o/centesis means tapping or puncture of the abdomen. This is a surgical puncture. The word for surgical puncture of the abdomen is ___abdomin /o /centesis___.

abdomin/o/centesis
abdominocentesis
ab dom′ i nō sen tē′ sis

426
Centesis (surgical puncture) is a word in itself. Build a word meaning surgical puncture, puncture, or tapping of the abdomen. ___abdominocentesis___

abdominocentesis

427
The unborn baby is protected by a sac (the amnion) filled with fluid. Tapping or puncturing this sac is called ___amni/o /centesis___.

amni/o/centesis
amniocentesis
am′ nē ō sen tē′ sis

428
The word for surgical puncture of the heart is ___cardi /o /centesis___.

cardi/o/centesis
cardiocentesis
kär′ dē ō sen tē′ sis

429

Abdomin/o/cyst/ic means pertaining to the abdomen and bladder. Analyze the word.

abdomin/o

cyst

ic
abdomin/o/cyst/ic
abdominocystic
ab dom' i nō sis' tik

_____ abdomin /o combining form

____ cyst ____ word root

__ ic __ suffix

Now put them together to form the word:
__ abdomin/o / cyst / ic __

Rework Review Sheets 1 and 2.

430

From abdomin/o/cyst/ic you see that the word root for bladder is __ cyst __.

431

cyst/o is used to form words that refer to the __ bladder __.

432

To refer to the urinary bladder, or **any sac containing fluid,** use some form of __ cyst /o __.

433

The word for incision into the bladder is
__ cyst / otomy __.

434

The word for excision of the bladder is
__ cyst / ectomy __.

435

A herniation of the bladder is a
__ cyst / o / cele __.

cyst/o/cele
cystocele
sis' tō sēl

436

When the bladder herniates into the vagina, a __ cystocele __ is formed.

437

Abdomin/o/thorac/ic means pertaining to the abdomen and thorax. The thorax is the chest. Analyze this word:

abdomin/o

thorac

ic

<u>abdomin o</u>   abdomen

<u>thorac</u>   thorax

<u>i e</u>   adjective—
     pertaining to

abdomin/o/thorac/ic
abdominothoracic
ab dom′ i nō thô ras′ ik

Now put them together to form

<u>abdomin/o/thorac/ic</u>.

438

Abdomin/o/thorac/ic pain means, literally, pain in the abdomen and chest. A physician who wants to say that there were lesions in these areas could

abdominothoracic

say <u>abdominothoracic</u>
lesions.

439

thorac/ic
thoracic
thô ras′ ik

thorac/o is used to form words about the thorax or chest. A word that means pertaining to the chest is <u>thorac / ic</u>. See the illustration of body cavities following Frame 440.

440

thorac/otomy
thoracotomy
thôr ə kot′ ə mē

A word that means incision of the chest is <u>thorac / otomy</u>.

441

thorac/o/centesis
thoracocentesis
thôr′ ə kō sen tē′ sis

A word that means surgical tapping of the chest to remove fluids is

<u>thorac /o / centesis</u>.

(surgical puncture)

442

thorac/o/path/y
thoracopathy
thôr ə kop′ ə thē

A word that means any chest disease is

<u>thorac/o / path / y</u>.

443

thorac/o/plast/y
thoracoplasty
thôr′ ə kō plas tē

A word for surgical repair of the chest is

<u>thorac /o/ plast / y</u>.

68

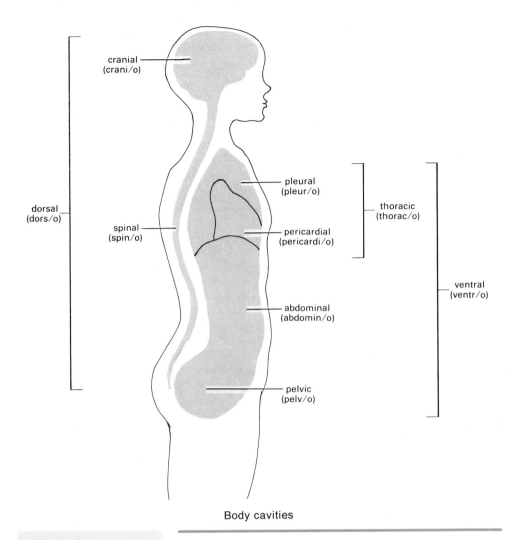

cranial
(crani/o)

pleural
(pleur/o)

thoracic
(thorac/o)

dorsal
(dors/o)

spinal
(spin/o)

pericardial
(pericardi/o)

ventral
(ventr/o)

abdominal
(abdomin/o)

pelvic
(pelv/o)

Body cavities

answer column	
cyst/o/plast/y cystoplasty sis′ tō plas tē	**444** A word for surgical repair of the bladder is _cyst / o / plast / y_.
water or fluid or watery fluid	**445** A hydr/o/cyst is a sac (or bladder) filled with watery fluid. Hydr/o is used in words to mean * _water or fluid_.
hydr/o/cephal/us hydrocephalus hī drō sef′ ə ləs	**446** Hydr/o/cephal/us is characterized by an enlarged head due to increased amount of fluid in the skull. A collection of fluid in the head is called _hydr / o / cephal / us_.

69

answer column

447

Hydrocephalus, unless arrested, results in deformity. The face seems small. The eyes are abnormal. The head is large. _hydrocephalus_

_____ also causes brain damage.

hydrocephalus

448

Because of the damage to the brain, children with _hydrocephalus_ are usually mentally retarded.

hydrocephalus

449

Hydrocephalus is the noun. The adjectival ending is ic. _hydr / o / cephal / ic_ children can be seen in schools for the mentally impaired.

hydr/o/cephal/ic
hydrocephalic
hī drō sə fal' ik

450

Hydr/o/phob/ia means having an abnormal fear of water. Phob/ia means
** _abnormal fear_ .

abnormal fear

451

Phob/ia is a word meaning any
** _abnormal fear_ .

abnormal fear

452

In a dictionary find the word phobia. How many phobias do you recognize already?
** _____. An abnormal fear of water is _hydr / o / phob / ia_.

between 3 and 12
hydr/o/phob/ia
hydrophobia
hī drō fō' bē ə

453

Some parents are abnormally afraid to have their children swim or even ride in a boat. These parents suffer from
hydro / phobia .

hydro/phobia

454

There is also a disease acquired from the bite of a rabid dog called
hydro phobia .

hydrophobia

70

455

Therap/y means treatment. Treatment by water is

hydr /o / therap / y .

hydr/o/therap/y
hydrotherapy
hī drō ther′ ə pē

456

Swirling water baths are a form of

hydro therapy .

hydrotherapy

✗ Work Review Sheets 5 and 6.

457

In words such as carcinoma and coccus, the first "**c**" is pronounced as a hard "**c**" or "**k**" sound. When followed by an "**o**" or "**a**" or a consonant, a "**c**" is pronounced like a "**k**" sound.

explanation for next frame

458

In the words colon and cardiac, the "**c**" is pronounced with a "__k__" sound.

hard "**c**" or "**k**"
(pronounce them aloud)

Listen to the cassette tapes that accompany this text for coaching on pronunciation.

459

In the words cerebrum and incision the "**c**" is pronounced as a soft or "**s**" sound. When "**c**" is followed by an "**i**" or "**e**" or "**y**", it is pronounced with a soft "**s**" sound.

explanation for next frame

460

According to the "**c**" rule, in the words cystocele and encephalitis each "**c**" is pronounced with a _____ sound.

soft or "**s**"

461

Remember the "**c**" rule for those terms that follow with all of their "**c**"s.

462

When building words about the spherically shaped family of bacteria, the cocc/i, use the word root _cocc_.

cocc

71

463

Pneumonia may be caused by pneumococcus. From this you know the bacteria responsible for pneumonia belongs to the family ___cocci___ (plural).

Disease-producing microorganisms

diplococcus

staphylococcus

streptococcus

typhoid bacillus

virus

spirochete

trichomonas

yeast

464

One form of meningitis is caused by the meningococcus. It, too, is a member of the family
___cocci___ (plural).

cocc/i

465

There are three main types of cocci.
Cocci growing in pairs are
___dipl / o / cocci___ .

dipl/o/cocc/i

72

answer column	

answer column

strept/o/cocc/i

staphyl/o/cocc/i

Cocci growing in twisted chains are
strept / o / _cocc_ / _i_ .

Cocci growing in clusters are
staphyl / o / _cocc_ / _i_ .

466

strept/o means twisted. Streptococci grow in twisted chains like this ∿∿∿ . If you should see a chain of cocci when examining a slide under the microscope, you would say they were

strept/o/cocc/i

strept / o / cocc / i .

467

Name the type of coccus in the following statements. Sore throat may be caused by B-hemolytic

strept/o/coccus

Strept / o / coccus. Some pus formation is due

Strept/o/coccus

to _Strept / o / coccus_ pyogenes. *Note:* Proper genus and species names are usually found italicized with genus capitalized. When using the genus initial it should also be capitalized. Examples: *Staphylococcus aureus*   *S. aureus*

468

"Staphyle" is the Greek word for **bunch of grapes.** **staphyl/o** is used to build words that suggest a bunch of grapes. Staphylococci grow in clusters like

grapes

a bunch of _grapes_ .

469

Staphylococci grow in clusters like grapes. If you should see a cluster of cocci when using the microscope, you would say they were

staphyl/o/cocc/i
staf i lō kok′ sī

staphyl / o / cocc / i .

470

The bacteria that cause carbuncles grow in a cluster like a bunch of grapes. Carbuncles are caused by

staphyl/o/cocc/i

staphyl / o / cocc / i .

471

Most bacteria that form pus grow in a cluster. They

staphylococci

are _staphylococci_ .

73

answer column	
staphylococci	**472** A common form of food poisoning is also caused by _staphylococci_.
staphyl/o	**473** At the back of the mouth, hanging like a bunch of grapes, is the uvula. To build words about the uvula you also use the word root—combining form that means **like a bunch of grapes.** This is _staphyl/o_.
staphyl/o/plast/y staphyloplasty staf' i lō plas tē	**474** Surgical repair of the uvula is _staphyl/o plast/y_.
inflammation of the uvula	**475** Staphyl/itis means ** _inflammation of th uvula_.
excision of the uvula	**476** Staphyl/ectomy means ** _excision of the uvula_.
uvul/o uvul/itis uvulitis ū vū lī′ tis uvul/ectomy uvulectomy ū vū lek′ tō mē	**477** **uvul/o** is also used when referring to, the palatine uvula. Build words meaning: inflammation of the uvula _uvula itis_ removal of the uvula _uvulectomy_
pus	**478** **py/o** is the word root—combining form used for words involving pus. A py/o/cele is a hernia containing _pus_.
pus	**479** Many staphylococci are pyogenic. Py/o/gen/ic means producing _pus_.
pus	**480** Py/orrhea means discharge of _pus_.

74

481

Py/o/thorax means an accumulation of pus in the thoracic cavity. When pus-forming bacteria invade the thoracic lining, _Py/o/thorax_ results.

py/o/thorax
pyothorax
pī ō thôr′ aks

482

Pyothorax may follow chest disease. Pneumonia is one chest disease that can result in _Py o thorax_.

483

Bronchopneumonia and bronchiectasis are two other diseases causing _pyothorax_.

484

A py/o/gen/ic bacterium is one that forms pus. You know the noun "genesis" for formation or beginning. The adjective that means something that produces or forms pus is _Py/o/gen/ic_.

py/o/gen/ic
pyogenic
pī ō jen′ ik

485

Pyogenic bacteria are found in boils. Boils become purulent (contain pus). This pus is formed by _pyogenic_ bacteria.

486

One type of staphylococcus causes boils. Therefore, you can say these staphylococci are _pyogenic_ bacteria.

487

orrhea is a combining form that you will use as a suffix. **orrhea** ends a word and it follows a word root. **orrhea** means flow or discharge. Py/orrhea means
** _pus flow, discharge_.

488

orrhea refers to any flow or discharge. A discharge or flow of pus is called _pyorrhea_.

75

answer column

489

Pyorrhea alveolaris is a disease of the teeth and gums. The part of this disease's name that tells you that pus is discharged is _pyorrhea_ .

pyorrhea

490

There is also a disease of the salivary gland symptomized by the flow of pus. This is _pyorrhea_ _____ salivaris.

pyorrhea

491

Ot/orrhea means a discharging ear. **ot/o** is the word root-combining form for _ear_ .

ear

492

Ot/orrhea is both a symptom and a disease. No matter which is meant, the word _Ot/orrhea_ is used.

ot/orrhea
otorrhea
ō tō re′ ə

493

The disease, otorrhea, involves discharge, inflammation, and deafness. One of the symptoms of this disease is found in its name, _otorrhea_ .

otorrhea

494

Otorrhea may be caused by ot/itis media. Ot/itis means

** _infla_ _____ .

inflammation of the ear

495

Otitis usually causes **ear pain,** which in medical terminology we call _ot/o/dyn/ia_

or _ot/algia_ .

ot/o/dyn/ia
ō tō din′ ē ə
ot/algia
ō tal′ jē ə

496

When otorrhea is established as a disease, there has been enough destruction of the tissue that _otodynia_ (ear pain) no longer occurs.

otodynia or
otalgia

76

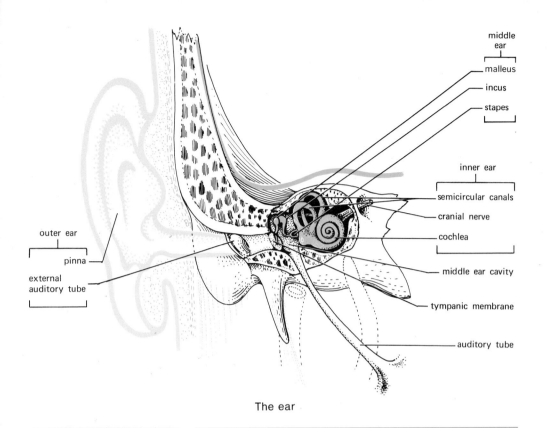

The ear

497

Small children often complain of earache. Medically, this could be called ___*otodynia*___ .

498

Look up **tympanum** in your dictionary. The tympanum is the ___*eardrum*___ . The word root–combining form for tympanum is ___*tympan/o*___ .

499

Build a word meaning:
  pertaining to the eardrum
    ___*tympan/ic*___

  incision into the eardrum
    ___*tympan/o/tomy*___

  excision of the eardrum
    ___*tympan/ectomy*___

tympan/ic
        /al
tim pan′ ik

tympan/otomy
tim pə not′ ə mē
tympan/ectomy
tim pə nek′ tə mē

77

answer column	
	500 In your dictionary, using the word root tympan, find a word that means **distended with gas**—as tight as a drum. The word is
tympanites tim pə nī′ tēz	_tympanites_ .
	501 Rhinorrhea means discharge from the nose. Rhin/o is used in words about the _nose_ .
nose	
	502 Using what is necessary from rhin/o, form a word that means inflammation of the nose.
rhin/itis rhinitis rī nī′ tis	_rhin/itis_
	503 Rhin/orrhea is a symptom. Drainage from the nose due to a head cold is a symptom called
rhin/orrhea rhinorrhea rī nə rē′ ə	_rhinorrhea_ .
	504 A discharge from the sinuses through the nose is a form of _rhinorrhea_ .
rhinorrhea	
	505 Nasal catarrh is another source of
rhinorrhea	_rhinorrhea_ .
rhin/o/plast/y rhinoplasty rī′ nō plas tē	**506** Build a word that means surgical repair of the nose. _rhin/o/plast/y_
rhin/otomy rhinotomy rī not′ ə mē	**507** Form a word that means incision of the nose. _rhin/otomy_
calculus or stone	**508** A rhin/o/lith is a calculus or stone in the nose. **lith/o** is the combining form for ** _calculus or stone_

78

Lithogenesis means producing or forming
** _calculi_ .

Lithology is the science of dealing with or studying
calculi .

Using what is necessary from lith/o, build a word meaning: an incision for the removal of a stone
lith /otomy ; an instrument for measuring size of calculi
lith /o/ meter .

Calculi or stones can be formed many places in the body. A chol/e/lith is a gallstone. **Chol/e** is the word root—combining form for _gall_ .

Chol/e/lith means gallstone. One cause of gall-bladder disease is the presence of a gallstone or
chol /e/ lith .

---

iasis is a suffix used to indicate a pathological condition. **iasis** is usually used when an infestation has occurred.

Lith/iasis is a disease condition in which a part of the body is infested by a stone. Infestation of the gallbladder with a gallstone is called:
chol /e/ lith/iasis

For the disease conditions stated below look up the cause of the infestation:

trichomoniasis _____

moniliasis _____

elephantiasis * _____

answer column

calculi (calculus)
or stones

calculi
or stones

lith/otomy
lithotomy
li thot' ə mē
lithometer
(You pronounce)

gall or bile

chol/e/lith
cholelith
kō′ lə lith

chol/e/lith/iasis
cholelithiasis
ko lē lith i′ ə sis

yeast (monilia)

trichomonas

nematode worm

517

Gall is secreted by the gallbladder. Chol/e/cyst is a medical name for the

_____.

gallbladder

518

Gallstones can result in inflammation of the gall-bladder (chol/e/cyst). Medically, this is called

_____/_____/_____/_____ .

chol/e/cyst/itis
cholecystitis
kō lə sis tī′ tis

519

Cholecystitis is accompanied by pain and hyper-emesis. Fatty foods aggravate these symptoms and should be avoided in cases of

_____.

cholecystitis

520

Butter, cream, and even whole milk contain fat and should be avoided by patients with

_____ .

cholecystitis

521

When a cholelith causes cholecystitis, one of two surgical procedures may be needed. One is an inci-sion into the gallbladder, a

_____/_____/_____/_____ .

chol/e/cyst/otomy
cholecystotomy
kō lə sis tot′ə mē
or
chol/e/lith/otomy
cholelithotomy
kō le li thot′ ə mē

522

Usually the presence of a gallstone calls for the excision of the gallbladder. This is a

_____/_____/_____/_____ .

chol/e/cyst/ectomy
cholecystectomy
kō lə sis tek′ tə mē

523

A calculus or stone in the nose is a

_____/_____/_____ .

rhin/o/lith
rhinolith
rī′ nō lith

524

How do you know **what** to put **where?** Following you will find material to assist you with word building. This is a system that you may have already figured out. If not, study these rules:

RULE 1: About 90 percent of the time, the part of the word that is indicated first comes last.

Examples

1. Inflammation of the bladder

inflammation	_____ / itis	
(of the) bladder	cyst / _____	
	cyst / itis	

2. One who specializes in skin disorders

one who specializes (studies)	_____ / / logist
(in) skin (disorders)	dermat / o / _____
	dermat / o / logist

3. Pertaining to the abdomen and bladder

pertaining to	_____ / / / ic
(the) abdomen	abdomin / o / _____ /
(and) bladder	_____ / / cyst /
	abdomin / o / cyst / ic

RULE II: Where body systems are involved, words are usually built in the order that organs are learned in the system.

Examples

1. Inflammation of the stomach and small intestine

inflammation	_____ / / / itis
(of the) stomach	gastr / o / _____ /
(and) small intestine	_____ / / enter /
	gastr / o / enter / itis

2. Removal of the uterus, fallopian tubes, and ovaries

removal of	_____ / / / / / ectomy
(the) uterus	hyster /o/ / / /
fallopian tubes	_____ / / salping /o/ /
(and) ovaries	_____ / / / / -oophor /
	hyster /o/ salping /o/ -oophor / ectomy

Of course, prefixes still come in front of the word.

---

answer column	525
slow	**brad/y** is used in words to mean slow. Brad/y/cardi/a means _____slow_____ heart action.

81

answer column	
brad/y/phag/ia bradyphagia brad i fā′ je ə	**526** Brad/y/phag/ia means slowness in eating. Abnormally slow swallowing is also called _brad/y/phag/ia_ .
bradyphagia	**527** From brad/y/phag/ia you find the word root **phag** for eat. (More of phag/o later.) Slow eating is _bradyphagia_ .
bradyphagia	**528** Children who play with their food while eating are exhibiting _bradyphagia_ .
brad/y/cardi/a bradycardia brad i kär′ dē ə	**529** Abnormally slow heart action is _brad/y/cardi/a_ .
fast or rapid	**530** **tach/y** is used in words to show the opposite of slow. tach/y means ** _fast or rapid_
rapid heart action	**531** Tach/y/cardi/a means ** _rapid heart action_
tach/y/phag/ia tachyphagia tak i fā′ jē ə	**532** The word for fast eating is _tach/y/phag/ia_ .
tachogram	**533** Tachos is a Greek word that means swiftness. A record of the velocity of the blood flow is a _tachogram_ .
tach/y/cardi/a tachycardia tak i kär′ dē ə	**534** An abnormally fast heartbeat is called _tach/y/cardi/a_ .
breathe or breathing	**535** **pne/o** comes from the Greek word pneia, breathe. **pne/o** any place in a word means _pne-o_ .

82

536

When pne/o begins a word, the "**p**" is silent. When pne/o occurs later in a word, it is pronounced. In pne/o/pne/ic the first "**p**" is _____ silent _____; the second is pronounced.

537

In pne/o/pne/ic, pne refers to _____ breathing _____.

538

Brad/y/pne/a means ** _____ bradypnea _____. A word for rapid breathing is _____ tach / y / pne / a _____.

slow breathing
tach/y/pne/a
tachypnea
tak ip nē′ ə

539

The rate of respiration (breathing) is controlled by the amount of carbon dioxide in the blood. Increased carbon dioxide speeds up breathing and causes _____ tachypnea _____.

540

Muscle exercise increases the amount of carbon dioxide in the blood. This speeds respiration and produces _____ tachypnea _____.

541

Running a race causes _____ tachypnea _____.

542

a is a prefix meaning **without.** Apnea literally means ** _____ without breathing _____.

543

A/pnea **really** means temporary cessation of breathing. If the failure to breathe were not temporary, death would result rather than _____ a / pne / a _____.

a/pne/a
apnea
ap nē′ ə, ap′ nē ə

544

Apnea means temporary cessation of breathing. If the level of carbon dioxide in the blood falls very low, _____ apnea _____ results.

83

answer column	

Answer column:

apnea
brad/y/pne/a
bradypnea
brad ip nē′ e

a

without generation (origin)

a/genes/is
agenesis
ə jen′ ə sis

agenesis

agenesis

carcin/o/genes/is
carcinogenesis
kar sin o jen′ sis

carcin/o/gen/ic
carcinogenic
kar sin o jen′ ic

dys/men/orrhea
dysmenorrhea
dis men ō rē′ a

545

When breathing ceases for a bit, _apnea_ results. If breathing is merely very slow, it is called _brad/y/pne/a_.

546

The prefix meaning **without** is _a_.

547

Genesis is both a Greek and an English word. It means generation (origin or beginning). A/genes/is means ** _without generation_.

548

By extension, agenesis means failure to develop or lack of development. When an organ does not develop, physicians use the word _a/genes/is_.

549

Agenesis can refer to any part of the body. If a hand does not develop, the condition is called _agenesis_ of the hand.

550

When the stomach is not formed, _agenesis_ of the stomach results.

551

The development of cancer is called _carcin/o/genes/is_.

552

A term that means pertaining to the development of cancer is _carcin/o/gen/ic_.

553

Dys is the prefix for painful, faulty, diseased, bad, or difficult. **Men** is the word root for menstruation.

554

Painful or difficult menstruation is _dys/men/orrhea_.

84

answer column	

555

Dysphagia means difficult swallowing. Analyze dysphagia. ___dys / phag / ia___

dys/phag/ia
dis fā′ jē ə

dys in dysphagia means

difficult
_____.

556

Dys/troph/y literally means bad development. The word for difficult breathing is

dys/pne/a
dyspnea
disp nē′

___dys / troph / y___.

557

pepsis is the Greek word for digestion. From this you get the word root–combining form peps/o to use in words about ___digestion___.

digestion

558

Dys/peps/ia means poor ___digestion___.
When food is eaten too rapidly,

digestion,
dys/peps/ia
dyspepsia
dis pep′ sh

___dys / peps / ia___ may result.

559

Dyspepsia is a noun. Eating under tension also causes ___dyspepsia___.

dyspepsia

560

Contemplating the troubles of the world when eating is a good cause for ___dyspepsia___.

dyspepsia

561

Cessation of digestion (without digestion) is

a/peps/ia   apepsia
a pep′ shə
brad/y/peps/ia
bradypepsia
brad i pep′ shə

___a / peps / ia___, while slow digestion
is ___brad / y / peps / ia___.

Work Review Sheets 8 and 9.

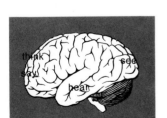

562

Refer to the chart on the next page when working Frames 563 through 583.

Information for working Frames 563 through 583.

COMBINING FORM	COMBINING FORM	SUFFIX
my/o (muscle)	spasm o/spasm/o (twitch, twitching)	spasm (word in itself)
	blast o/blast/o (germ or embryonic; gives rise to something else)	blast (word in itself)
angi/o (vessel)	scler/o (hard)	osis (use with scler/o)
	fibr/o (fibrous, fiber)	oma (use with fibr/o)
neur/o (nerve or neuron)	lys/o (breaking down, destruction)	is—noun suffix (use with lys/o)

answer column

563

An embryonic (germ) cell from which a muscle cell develops is a **my/o/blast**.

A germ cell from which a nerve cell develops is a

neur/o/blast
noor′ ō blast

_____ neuro / o / blast .

A germ cell from which vessels develop is an

angi/o/blast
an′ jē o blast

angi / o / blast .

564

A spasm of a nerve is a **neur/o/spasm**.

my/o/spasm
mī′ ō spaz əm

A spasm of a muscle is a _____ my / o / spasm .

A spasm of a vessel is an

angi/o/spasm
an′ jē ō spaz əm

angi / o / spasm .

565

A (condition of) hardening of nerve tissue is **neur/o/scler/osis**.

A hardening of a vessel is

angi/o/scler/osis
an jē ō sklə rō′ sis

angi / o / scler / osis

A hardening of muscle tissue is

my/o/scler/osis
mī′ ō sklə rō′ sis

my / o / scler / osis .

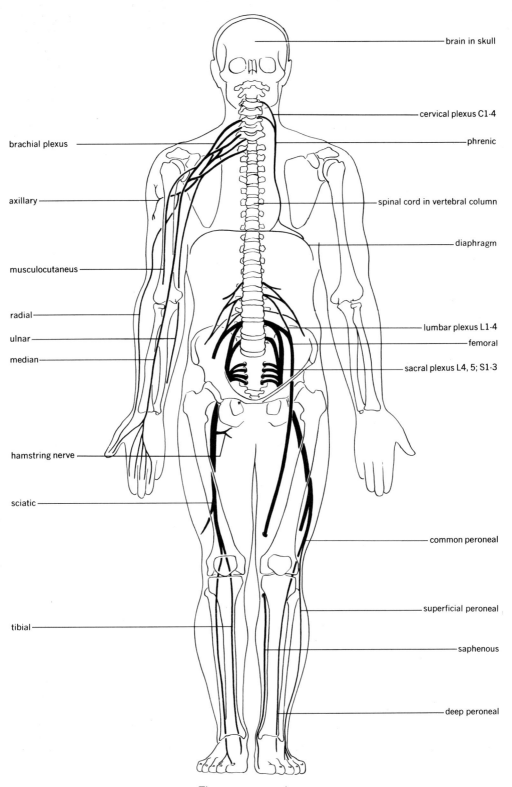

brain in skull

cervical plexus C1-4

phrenic

brachial plexus

spinal cord in vertebral column

axillary

diaphragm

musculocutaneus

radial

lumbar plexus L1-4

ulnar

femoral

median

sacral plexus L4, 5; S1-3

hamstring nerve

sciatic

common peroneal

superficial peroneal

tibial

saphenous

deep peroneal

The nervous system

answer column

566

A tumor containing muscle fibers is a **my/o/fibr/oma.**

A tumor containing nerve fibers is a

neur/o/fibr/oma
noor ō fī brō′ mə

neur /o/ fibr / oma

A vessel tumor containing fibers is an

angi/o/fibr/oma
an′ jē o fī bro′ mə

angi /o/ fibr / oma

567

The destruction of muscle tissue is **my/o/lys/is.**

The destruction of nerve tissue is

neur/o/lys/is
noo rol′ ə sis

neur /o/ lys /is.

The destruction or breaking down of vessels is

angi/o/lys/is
an jē ol′ əs is

angi /o/ lys /is.

568

Arteri/o is used in words about the arteries. Arteries are blood vessels that carry blood away from the heart. A word meaning **hardening of the arteries is**

arteri/o/scler/osis
arteriosclerosis
är tir′ ē ō sklə rō′ sis

arteri/o / scler /osis.

569

Arteri/o/scler/osis means hardening of the arteries. Build a word meaning:

a fibrous condition of the arteries

arteri/o/fibr/osis
är tir′ ē ō fī brō′ sis

arteri/o / fibr / osis;

a softening of the arteries

arteri/o/malac/ia
är tir′ ē ō mə lā′ shə

arteri/o / malac / ia.

570

Give a word for:

arterial spasm

arteri/o/spasm
är tir′ ē ō spaz əm

arteri/o /spasm;

gastric spasm

gastr/o/spasm
gas′ trō spaz əm
gastr/o/malac/ia
gas trō mə lā′ shə

gastr /o /spasm;

softening of the stomach walls

gastr /o / malac / ia.

88

answer column	

Build a word meaning:

destruction (breakdown) of fat

lip/o/lys/is
li pol′ ə sis

lip / o / lys / is ;

destruction (breakdown) of cells

cyt/o/lys/is
sī tol′ ə sis

cyt / o / lys / is .

572

hem/o refers to blood. A tumor of a blood vessel is
a hem/angi/oma. (Note dropped **o**.)
An inflammation of a blood vessel is

hem/angi/itis
hē man jē ī′ tis
hem/arthr/osis
hē mär thrō′ sis,
hem är thrō′ sis

hem / angi / itis .

A condition of blood in a joint is

hem / arthr / osis .

573

hemat/o also refers to blood.
Another word for destruction of blood tissue is

hemat/o/lys/is
hē mə tol′ ə sis,
hem ə tol′ ə sis
hemat/o/phob/ia
hē mə tō fō′ bē ə,
hem e to fō′ be e

hemat / o / lys / is .

Phobia means fear.
An abnormal fear of blood is

hemat / o / phob / ia .

574

blood
hemat/o/log/y
hē mə tol′ ə je,
hem ə tol′ ə jē
hemat/o/log/ist
hē mə tol′ ə jist,
hem ə tol′ ə jist

Still use hemat/o to mean _blood_ .
The study of blood is

hemat / o / logy / .

One who specializes in the science of blood is a

hemat / o / log / ist .

575

thromb/o is the word root-combining form that
means clot. Thromb/o/angi/itis means inflammation of a vessel with formation of a _clot_

clot

.

576

excision of a
thrombus (clot).

Thromb/ectomy means ** _excision of a clot_ .

89

577

The proper medical way to say clot is to say throm-bus. A synonym for clot is ___*thrombus*___.

thrombus

---

inflammation of a lymph
vessel with formation
of a thrombus (clot) or
a condition of this

578

Thromb/o/lymph/angi/itis means **_____

_____.

579

Thromb/o/phleb/itis means **_____

inflammation of a vein
with thrombus formation

_____.

580

Using thromb/o, build a word meaning:
  a condition of forming a thrombus

thrombosis
throm bō' sis

_____ / _____ ;

  a cell that aids clotting

thrombocyte
throm' bō sīt

_____ / ___ / _____ ;

  resembling a thrombus

thromboid
throm' boid

_____ / _____ .

581

Build a word meaning:
  pertaining to the formation of a thrombus

thromb/o/gen/ic
throm bō jen' ik

_____ / ___ / _____ ;

  destruction of a thrombus

thromb/o/lysis
throm bol' ə sis

_____ / ___ / _____ ;

  lack of cells that aid clotting

thromb/o/cyt/o/penia
throm bō sī tō pē' nē ə

_____ / ___ / _____ / ___ / _____ .

---

formation of spermatozoa
or
formation of sperm
or
formation of male germ
cells

582

Sperma is the Greek word meaning seed. **spermat/o**
is used in words about spermat/o/zoa or male germ
cells (sperm), Spermat/o/genesis means
**_____

_____.

Give a word meaning:
    the destruction of spermatozoa

____ / ____ / _____ / _____ ;

an embryonic male cell

____ / ____ / _____ .

A bladder or sac containing sperm is a

_____ / ____ / _____ .

A word for resembling sperm is

_____ / _____ .

A word for disease of sperm is

_____ / ____ / _____ / ____ .

Summarize what you learned in Frames 563 to 570.

    my/o   means _____ .

    angi/o   means _____ .

    neur/o   means _____ .

    spasm   means _____ .

    blast/o   means _____ .

    scler/o   means _____ .

    fibr/o   means _____ .

    lys/o   means _____ .

    thromb/o   means _____ .

    spermat/o   means _____ .

    hemat/o   means _____ .

    hem/o   means _____ .

    genesis   means _____ .

Orchid/algia means pain in the testicle. Orchid/
ectomy means *_____
_____ .

---

answer column

spermat/o/lys/is
spûr mə tol′ ə sis

spermat/o/blast
spûr mat′ ō blast

spermat/o/cyst
spûr ma′ ō sist

spermat/oid
spûr′ mə toid

spermat/o/path/y
spûr mə top′ ə thē

muscle

vessel

nerve

twitching

germ or embryonic

hard

fibrous

destruction

clot

spermatozoa (sperm)

blood

blood

formation

excision of a testicle

589

Around the time of birth the testicles normally descend from the abdominal cavity into the scrotum. Sometimes this fails to happen (crypt/orchid/ism). Surgical repair is indicated. The operation is called an

_____ / ___ / _____ / _____ .

orchid/o/plast/y
orchidoplasty
 r' ki dō plas tē

590

Build a word meaning:
   herniation near a testicle

_____ / ___ / _____ ;

   incision into a testicle

_____ / ___ / _____ ;

The male reproductive system

591

Crypt/orchid/ism means undescended testicle. **Crypt** means hidden. When a testicle is hidden in the abdominal cavity, the condition is known as

_____ / ___ / _____ .

crypt/orchid/ism
cryptorchidism
krip tôr' ki diz əm

592

A crypt/ic remark is one with a hidden meaning. A crypt/ic belief is one whose meaning is

_____.

593

A crypt/o/gram is writing in code. Crypt/o/toxic means having toxins (poisons) whose action is

_____.

594

A crypt is a hidden gland or follicle. Build a word meaning:

inflammation of a crypt

_____ / _____ ;

excision of a crypt

_____ / _____ .

595

When an organ contains pus that is concealed (hidden), it is said to be

crypt / o / py / ic .

596

Excessive secretion (flow) of an endocrine (hidden) gland is called

crypt / orrhea .

597

The Greek word for egg is oon. In scientific words, o/o (pronounce both o's) means egg or ovum. An o/o/blast is

** emb. egg .

an embryonic egg cell
(a cell that will become
an ovum)

598

O/o/genesis is the formation and development of an ovum. The changes that occur in the cell from ooblast to mature ovum are

_____ / _____ / _____ .

o/o/genesis
oogenesis
ō ə jen′ ə sis

599

Oogenesis must be complete for the ovum to be mature. It is impossible for a spermatozoon to fertilize an ovum until _____ is complete.

oogenesis

600

The word root—combining form used in words that refer to the ovary is **oophor/o.** When you see oophor in a word, you think of the _____.

ovary

601

The ovary is the organ that is responsible for maturing and discharging the ovum. About every 28 days an ovum is discharged from the

_____ovary_____.

ovary

602

This frame shows the development of oophorectomy:

o/o		egg	from Greek, oon
phor/o		bear	from Greek, phoros
ect/o		out	from Greek, ektos
tom/y	cut	from Greek, tomos

This is included for those who are interested.

603

oophor/o is used in words to refer to the ovary. Oophorectomy means

** _____ovary removed excision_____.

excision of the ovary

604

Using what you need from oophor/o, build a word that means:

inflammation of an ovary

_____oophor/itis_____;

excision of an ovary

_____oophor/ectomy_____;

tumor of an ovary
(ovarian tumor)

_____oophor/oma_____.

oophor/itis oophoritis
ō ə fə rī′ tis
oophor/ectomy
oophorectomy
ō ə fə rek′ tə mē
oophor/oma oophoroma
ō ə fə rō′ mə

94

answer column	
fixation	**605** Oophoropexy means fixation of a displaced ovary. Pex/y is a combining form that means _____fixation_____.
oophor/o/pex/y oophoropexy ō of′ ə rō pek sē	**606** An oophor/o/pex/y is a surgical procedure. When an ovary is displaced, an ___oophor / o / pex / y___ is performed.
oophoropexy	**607** Oophoropexy is a noun. You can see the noun suffix "y" ending the word ___oophor / o / pex / y___.
oophoropexy	**608** The surgical procedure for a prolapsed (dropped or sagged) ovary is called an ___oophoropexy___.
pexy	**609** In the male, fixation of a prolapsed testicle is called orchid/o/pexy. The suffix that means fixation is ___pexy___.
fallopian tube(s)	**610** **salping/o** is used to build words that refer to the fallopian tube(s). A salpingoscope is an instrument used to examine the *___fallopian tube___.
fallopian tube	**611** A salpingostomy is a surgical opening into a *___fallopian tub___.
salping/itis salpingitis sal pin jī′ tis salping/ectomy salpingectomy sal pin jek′ tə mē	**612** Using what you need of salping/o, build a word meaning: inflammation of a fallopian tube ___salping / itis___; excision of a fallopian tube ___salpingectomy___.

95

613

When you are building compound medical words and use two like vowels between word roots or combining forms, separate them with a hyphen. For a model use **salpingo-oophorectomy,** and build a word that means inflammation of the fallopian tube and ovary.

salping/o-/oophor/itis
salpingo-oophoritis
sal ping′ gō ō ə fə rī′ tis

salpingo /o /oophor /itis

614

A hernia that encloses the ovary and fallopian tube is a

salping/o-/oophor/o/cele
salpingo-oophorocele
sal ping′ gō ō of′ ə rō sēl

salping /o /oophor /o/ cele.

615

colp/o is used in words about the vagina. Colpitis means

inflammation of the
 vagina

* _____*inflammation vagina*_____.

616

Colp/o/dynia means ** *vaginal pain*

vaginal pain
colp/o/path/y
colpopathy
kol pop′ ə thē

_____. Any disease of the vagina is called

colp /o/ path /y.

617

A colp/o/spasm is a ** _____

vaginal spasm
colp/ectomy
colpectomy
kol pek′ tə mē

_____. Excision of a part of the vagina is a

colp /ectomy.

618

Build a word meaning:
 fixation of the vagina

colpopexy

colp /o/ pex /y;

 surgical repair of the vagina

colpoplasty
(You pronounce)

colp /o/ plasty.

619

Build a word meaning:
 instrument for examining the vagina

colposcope

colp /o/ scope /;

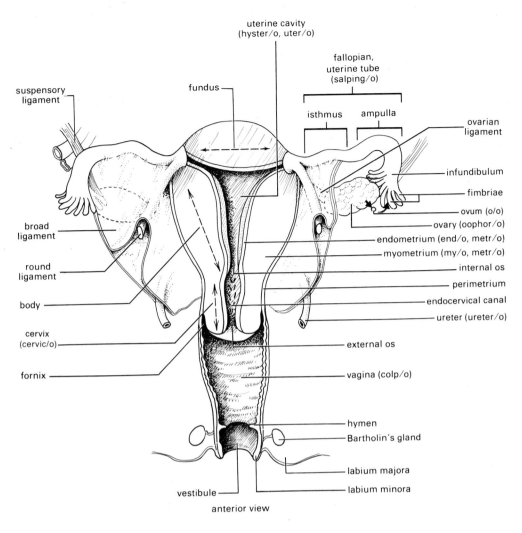

uterine cavity
(hyster/o, uter/o)

fallopian,
uterine tube
(salping/o)

isthmus   ampulla

fundus

suspensory
ligament

ovarian
ligament

infundibulum

fimbriae

ovum (o/o)

ovary (oophor/o)

broad
ligament

endometrium (end/o, metr/o)

myometrium (my/o, metr/o)

internal os

round
ligament

perimetrium

endocervical canal

ureter (ureter/o)

body

cervix
(cervic/o)

external os

fornix

vagina (colp/o)

hymen

Bartholin's gland

labium majora

vestibule

labium minora

anterior view

The femal reproductive system

incision into the vagina

$colp$ / $otomy$.

620
In words built from laryng/o, pharyng/o, salping/o,
and mening/o, the ''**g**'' is pronounced as a hard ''**g**''
when followed by an ''**o**'' or an ''**a.**'' The ''**g**'' in **good**
is a hard ''g.''

97

answer column

621

In laryngalgia and salpingocele, the "**g**" of the word root is pronounced hard as in "game." In pharyngalgia and meningocele, the word-root "g" also is given a _____ pronunciation.

hard
(Pronounce them)

622

In laryngostomy, pharyngotomy, salpingopexy, and meningomalacia, the "**g**" is given a _____ sound.

hard
(Pronounce them)

623

A hard "**g**" precedes the vowels _____ and _____.

o and a

624

In words built from laryng/o, pharyng/o, salping/o, and mening/o, the "**g**" is soft when followed by an "**e**" or an "**i.**" The "**g**" in **germ** and **giant** is soft.

explanation for next
 frame

625

In laryngectomy and salpingitis, the "**g**" is a soft "**g**" as in germ. In meningeal and pharyngitis, the "**g**" also is given a _____ pronunciation.

soft
(Pronounce them)

626

In meningitis, salpingian, laryngitis, and pharyngectomy, the "**g**" is given a _____ sound.

soft
(Pronounce them)

627

A soft "**g**" precedes the vowels _____ and _____.

e and i

628

"**g**" is given a hard sound when followed by the vowels _____ and _____. "**g**" is given the soft "**j**" sound when followed by the vowels _____ and _____.

a and o
e and i

629

In compound words a hyphen (-) is used when
** _____.

two like vowels join
 word roots or combining
 forms

630

The spermatozoon is the male germ cell; the ovum, the female egg cell. When they unite in the fallopian tube, conception has occurred. The fertilized ovum moves to the uterus, is implanted into the endometrium and is incubated until birth.

631
hyster/o is used to build words about the uterus. A hyster/ectomy is an excision of the _____ uterus .

uterus

632
A hysterotomy is an incision into the _____ uterus, and a hysterospasm is a spasm of the _____ uterus.

uterus

uterus

633
Hyster/o/pex/y means surgical fixation of the uterus. Any uterine disease is called

_____ hyster /o /path y

hyster/o/path/y
hysteropathy
his ter op′ ə thē

634
A hyster/o/salping/o-/oophor/ectomy is the excision of the uterus, fallopian tubes, and ovaries. Analyze this word:

_____ hyster /o combining form for uterus

_____ salping /o combining form for fallopian tubes

_____ oophor word root for ovary

_____ ectomy suffix–excision

hyster/o

salping/o

oophor
ectomy

635
hyster/o is used in words pertaining to the uterus; **metr/o** refers to the tissues of the same organ.

See ''Case Study: Gynecology Consultation'' on the opposite page.

636
hyster/o usually refers to the uterus as an organ. **metr/o usually** refers to the tissues of the _____ uterus.

uterus

99

---

organ tissues	**637** There are exceptions to the rule, but in general hyster/o means the uterus as an __organ__. Metr/o refers to the uterus in the sense of its __tissue__.
uterus or uterine musculature	**638** Metr/itis means an inflammation of the uterine musculature. Metr/o/paralysis means paralysis of the ** __uterine tissue__.
metr/orrhea mē trō rē′ ə, met rō rē′ ə	**639** Using metr/orrhagia as an example, build a word meaning flow or discharge from the uterine tissues __metr/orrhea__,

metr/o/path/y or
hysteropathy
metr/o/cele or
hysterocele
(You pronounce)
	640
	Build a word meaning:
	  any uterine disease
	  _____/ / /;
	  herniation of the uterus
	  _____/ /

641

The end/o/metr/ium is the lining of the uterus. Build a word meaning:

inflammation of the uterine lining

end / o / metr / itis ;

disease of the uterus

_____ / _____ / _____ .

---

hyster/o/salping/o-/
  oophor/ectomy
hysterosalpingo-
  oophorectomy
his′ tə rō salping′ gō-
ō ə fə rek′ tə mē

642

Build the word that means excision of the uterus, fallopian tubes, and ovaries.

hyster / o / salping / o / oophor / ectomy

643

A word meaning fixation of the uterus is

hyster / o / pex / y . A

word meaning uterine hernia is

hyster / o / cele .

hyster/o/pex/y
hysteropexy
his′ tə rō pek sē
hyster/o/cele
hysterocele
his′ tə rō sēl

644

optosis is a suffix meaning prolapse or downward displacement.

645

Hyster/o/ptosis means prolapse of the uterus. Ptosis is a word that means

prolapse .

646

Hysteroptosis is a compound word constructed from:

hyster/o the combining form for uterus;

ptosis a word meaning pro-lapse.

647

When prolapse occurs, a fixation is usually done. A hysteropexy would be done to correct or repair

hyster / o / ptosis .

hyster/o/ptosis
hysteroptosis
his tər op tō′ sis

101

648

Many organs can prolapse or sag. When the uterus prolapses, it is called

hysteroptosis

_____ .

649

When the broad ligament that helps support the uterus weakens,

hysteroptosis

_____

can occur.

---

colp/o/ptosis
colpoptosis
kol pop tō′ sis

650

Build a word meaning prolapse of the vagina.

Colp / o / ptosis

651

gynec/o comes from the Greek word "gyne," which means woman. The field of medicine called gyne-

women

cology deals with diseases of _women_ .

---

gynec/o/log/ist
gynecologist
gī nə kol′ ə jist,
jin ə kol′ ə jist

652

Gynec/o/log/ic or gynec/o/log/ical are adjectival forms of gynecology. The physician who specializes in female disorders is called a

gynec / o / logist .

653

Build a word meaning:
   resembling woman

gynecoid
gī′ nə koid, jin′ ə koid
gynecopathy
gī nə kop′ ə thē,
jin ə kop′ ə thē
gynecophobia
gī nə kō fō′ bē ə,
jin ə kō fō′ bē ə

   gynec / oid ;

any disease peculiar to women

   gynec / o / path / y ;

abnormal fear of women

   gynec / o / phob / i a .

Work Review Sheets 10 and 11.

102

nephr/o/ptosis nephroptosis nef rop tō′ sis	**654** **nephr/o** is used in words to refer to the kidney. A word that means prolapse of the kidney is _nephr / o / ptosis_ .
nephroptosis	**655** Nephr/o/ptosis can occur from a hard blow or jolt. People who ride motorcycles often wear special clothing or a kidney belt to protect against _nephroptosis_ .
inflammation of a kidney nephr/o/pex/y nephropexy nef′ rō pek sē nephr/o/lys/is nef rol′ ə sis	**656** Nephritis means ** _inflam. kidne_ . Build a word meaning: fixation of a kidney _nephr / o / pex / y_ ; destruction of kidney tissue _nephr / o / lys / is_ .
nephr/o/lith nef′ rō lith nephr/o/malac/ia nef rō mə lā′ shə nephr/o/megal/y nef rō meg′ ə lē	**657** Build a word meaning: stone in the kidney _nephr / o / lith_ ; softening of kidney tissue _nephr / o / malac / ia_ ; enlargement of the kidney _nephr / o / megaly_ .
ur	**658** **Ur**ology is the study of the **ur**inary tract. The **ur**inary tract is responsible for forming **ur**ine from waste materials in the blood, and eliminating **ur**ine from the body. What would you guess to be the word root for **ur**ine? _ur / o_ . (See illustration of urinary tract opposite Frame 660.)
renal pelvis	**659** **pyel/o** refers to the * _renal pelvis_ .

103

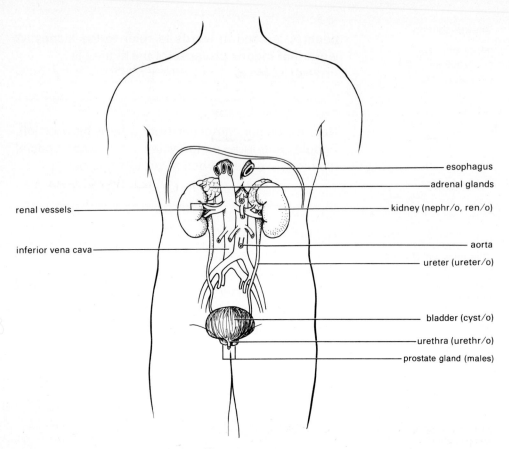

The urinary system

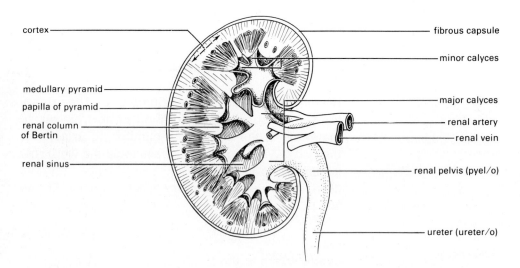

The kidney

Using what you need from the combining form for renal pelvis, form words meaning:
inflammation of the renal pelvis

_____ / _____ ;

surgical repair of the renal pelvis

pyel / o / plast / y.

WORD	WORD ROOT–COMBINING FORM	NEW SUFFIX TO USE WHEN NEEDED
urine	ur/o	
kidney	nephr/o	orrhaphy (suturing or stitching)
renal pelvis	pyel/o	orrhagia
ureter	ureter/o	(hemorrhage or "bursting forth" of blood)
bladder	cyst/o	
urethra	urethr/o	

661

Pyel/o/nephr/osis means ** _____
_____. Form a word that means inflammation of the renal pelvis and kidney.

pyel / o / nephr / itis

662

Ureter/o/lith means
** _____.

Form a word that means:
 herniation of the ureter

ureter / o / cele ;

any disease of the ureter

ureter / o / path y.

663

Ureter/o/pyel/o/plast/y means ** _____
_____.

Form a word meaning inflammation of the ureter and renal pelvis.

ureter / o / pyel / itis

answer column

664

Form a word meaning:

    making a new opening between the ureter and bladder

ureter/o/cyst/ostomy
yoo rē′ tə rō sis tos′
  tə mē

ureter / / cyst / ostomy ;

    a condition of the ureter involving pus

ureter/o/py/osis
yoo rē′ tə rō pī ō′ sis

ureter / o / py / osis .

665

Ureter/orrhaphy introduces a new word part. **orrhaphy** is not really a suffix, but again (for simplification) it can be used as one. orrhaphy means

suturing or stitching

** *suture* .

666

Form the word that means suturing of the ureter.

ureter/orrhaphy
ureterorrhaphy
yoo rē tə rôr′ ə fē

uter / orrhapy

667

Form a word meaning:

    suturing of a kidney

nephr/orrhaphy
nephrorrhaphy
nef rôr′ ə fē
cyst/orrhaphy
cystorrhaphy
sis tôr′ ə fē

nephr / orrhapy ;

    suture of the bladder

cyst / orrhapy .

668

Form a word meaning:

    suture of a nerve

neur/orrhaphy
noo rôr′ ə fē

neur / orrhapy ;

    suturing of the eyelids

blephar/orrhaphy
blef ə rôr′ ə fē

/ ;

    suturing of the vagina

colp/orrhaphy
kol pôr′ ə fē

colp / orrhapy .

669

carries urine from the
  body or removes urine
  from the bladder

urethr/o

The urethra is the organ that ** _____
_____. The word root–
combining form for urethra is

urethra / .

answer column

suturing of the urethra

urethr/otomy
yoor ə throt' ə mē

urethr/o/spasm
yoo rē' thrō spaz əm

urethra

urethr/o/cyst/itis
urethrocystitis
yoo rē' thrō sis tī' tis

hemorrhage or bursting
forth of blood

hemorrhage
urethr/orrhagia
urethrorrhagia
yoo rē thrō rā' jē ə

cyst/orrhagia
sis tə rā' jē ə

ureter/orrhagia
yoo rē' tə rō ra' jē ə

bladder

vesic/o

670

Urethr/orrhaphy means
** _suture of urethra_ .

Form a word meaning:
incision into the urethra

urethr / otomy ;

spasm of the urethra

urethr / o / spasm .

671

Urethr/o/rect/al means pertaining to the urethra and rectum. Urethr/o/vagin/al means pertaining to the _____ and vagina. Form a word that means inflammation of urethra and bladder.

urethr / o / cyst / itis .

672

orrhagia is another complex word part that can be used as a suffix because it follows a word root and ends a word. orrhagia means ** _hemorrage_
_____ .

673

Gastr/orrhagia means stomach hemorrhage. Encephal/orrhagia means brain _hemm._ .
A word that means hemorrhage of the urethra is
urethr / orrhagia .

674

Build a word meaning:
hemorrhage of the bladder

cyst / orrhagia ;

hemorrhage of the ureter

ureter / orragia .

675

Look up **vesica**, vesicle. They mean
_____ . Their word root–combining form is _vesica / o_ .

107

676

Look up **ren** (pl. renes). They mean

_____. Their word root–combining

form is ___ren /o___ .

677

Build a word meaning:

pertaining to the bladder

___vesic/al___ ;

herniation of a bladder

___vesic/o/cele___ ;

irrigation (washing) of a bladder

___vesic/o/clys/is___ .

vesic/al
ves' i kəl
vesic/o/cele
ves' i kō sēl

vesic/o/clys/is
ves i kok' lə sis
(cyst/o words
are correct.)

678

Build a word meaning:

pertaining to the kidney

___ren/al___ ;

any kidney disease

___ren/o/pathy___ ;

record from x-ray of the kidney

___ren/o/gram___ .

ren/al
rē' nəl
ren/o/path/y
re nop' ə thē
ren/o/gram

(You pronounce)

679

Renointestinal means

** _____.

Renogastric means

** _____.

680

Notice how these word roots were built from each other.

COMBINING FORM	MEANING	MEDICAL TERM
pne/o	breathing	tachy**pne**a
pneum/o	air	**pne**umothorax
pneumon/o	lung	**pne**umonectomy

681

pne/o refers to breathing. The lungs are the organs of the body that take in air (breathe). **Pne**umon/o is used in medical words concerning lungs. Pneumon/ectomy means

excision of lungs

**_____.

Incision of a lung is a

pneumon/otomy
nōō mə not′ ə mē

_____/_____.

682

Pneumon/o/path/y means

any disease of the lungs
pneumon/orrhagia
pneumonorrhagia
nōō′ mə nō rā′ jē ə

**_____.

Form a word meaning hemorrhage of a lung.

_____/_____.

683

Pneumonia is an acute inflammation of the lungs caused by a variety of organisms and viruses. Antibiotics are most used to treat pneumonia. Another word for pneumonia is pneumonitis.

684

Form a word meaning surgical puncture of a lung.

pneumon/o/centesis
nōō′ mə nō sen tē′ sis

_____/____/_____.

685

There are two words meaning inflammation of the lungs:

pneumon/ia
nōō mōn′ y ə

_____/_____

and

pneumon/itis
nōō mə nī′ tis

_____/_____.

686

Fixation of lung tissues to the chest wall is called

pneumon/o/pex/y
nōō′ mə nō pek sē

_____/____/____/_____.

687

Pneumon/o/melan/osis is a lung disease in which lung tissue becomes black due to breathing black dust. The word root for black is _____.

melan

688

Pneumon/o/melan/osis literally means a condition of black lungs. Analyze this word.

pneumon/o
_____/ combining form for lung

melan
_____ word root for black

osis
_____ suffix—condition

689

Construct a word meaning condition of lung blackness.

pneumon/o/melan/osis
pneumonomelanosis
nōō′ mə nō mel ə nō′ sis
_____

690

The inhalation (breathing) of black dust results in

pneumon/o/melan/osis
_____/ _____/ _____/ _____.

The inhalation of much soot or black smoke can

pneumonomelanosis
also cause _____.

691

black
melan/o means _____.

Melan/osis means black pigmentation. A word that

melan/oma
melanoma
mel ə nō′ mə
means black tumor is

_____/ _____.

692

Melan/in is the pigment that gives dark color to the hair, skin, and choroid of the eye. A black pigmented cell is a

melan/o/cyte
melanocyte
mel′ ə nō sīt
mə lan′ ə sīt
_____/ _____/ _____.

693

Melanoderma means

black or dark skin
coloring (pigmentation)
(literally—black skin)
** _____.

694

You have already learned that a carcin/oma is a form of cancer. A darkly pigmented cancer is

melan/o/carcin/oma
melanocarcinoma
mel′ ə nō kar si nō′ mə
_____/ _____/ _____/ _____.

695

Whenever any hairless mole on the skin turns black and grows, a physician should be consulted, for there is possible danger of black-mole cancer or

melanocarcinoma

_____.

696

Pneumon/o/myc/osis means a fungus disease of the lungs. The word root that means "fungus" is

myc

_____.

fungus (singular)
fung′ gəs
fungi (plural)
fun′ jī, fung′ gī

697

myc/o seen any place in a word should make you think of _____.

698

In high school biology, you read or even learned the words **myc**elium and **myc**elial. Myc refers

fungi or fungus

_____.

pneumon/o/myc/osis
pneumonomycosis
no͞o′ mə no͞ mī kō′ sis

699

A mycosis is any condition caused by a fungus. A condition of lung fungus is

_____ / ___ / ___ / _____.

700

myc/oid
mī′ koid
myc/o/log/y
mycology
mī kol′ ə jē

Build a word meaning:

resembling fungi _myc/o/id_____;

study of fungi _myc/o/log/y_____.

701

Build a word meaning:
fungus disease (condition) of the pharynx

pharyng_o/ myc/ osis;

pharyng/o/myc/osis
rhin/o/myc/osis
dermat/o/myc/osis
(Try to pronounce
them yourself)

fungus disease (condition) of the nose

rhin /o/ myc / osis;

fungus disease of the skin

derm/o/ myc /osis.

111

702

Pneum/o and pneumon/o can both refer to the lung. Pneum/o is derived from the Greek word "pneuma" (air). Pneum/o is used in words to mean air.

703

pneumono

lung or lungs

pneum/o comes from the Greek word "pneumon" (lung). **pneumon/o** is used in words that refer to the _____. The lungs are shown in the illustration for Frame 1290.

704

air

pneum/o comes from the Greek word "pneuma" (air). Pneum/o is used in most words to mean ___air___ but can also be used to mean lung.

705

pneum/o/thorax
pneumothorax
nōō mō thôr' aks

Your use of **pneum/o** will be in words about air. Pneum/o/derm/a means a collection of air under the skin. A collection of air in the chest cavity (thorax) is a

_____ / _____ / _____ .

706

thorac/o

pneum/o/thorac/ic
pneumothoracic

The word root-combining form for thorax (chest cavity) is _____ / _____. The adjective that pertains to a collection of air in the chest cavity is

_____ / _____ / _____ / _____ .

707

pneum/o/therap/y
pneumotherapy
nōō mō ther' ə pē

Hydrotherapy means treatment with water. Treatment with compressed air is called

_____ / _____ / _____ / _____ .

708

pneum/o/meter
nōō mom' ə tər

A tach/y/meter measures speed of any body in motion. An instrument that measures air volume in respiration is a

_____ / _____ / _____ .

112

709

A collection of air and serum in the chest cavity is pneum/o/ser/o/thorax. A collection of air and pus in the thoracic cavity is a

pneum/o/ py /o/ thorax,

while a collection of air and blood in this same cavity is a

pneum/o/ hem/o/ thorax

pneum/o/py/o/thorax
pneum/o/hem/o/thorax
(hemat/o/)
(You try the pronunciation yourself)

Work Review Sheets 12 and 13.   ✱ test #1

710

The illustration and information that follow will be used for building words through Frame 761.

ORGAN	WORD ROOT COMBINING FORM FOR ORGAN	ANOTHER WORD ROOT COMBINING FORM	
mouth	stomat/o		
teeth	dent/o		
tongue	gloss/o	clysis—washing or irrigation	
lips	cheil/o	(word in itself)	
gums	gingiv/o		
esophagus	esophag/o		
stomach	gastr/o		
small intestine	enter/o	ectasia—dilatation or stretching	
		(word in itself)	
duodenum (1st part)	duoden/o		
		combining form	**suffix**
large intestine or colon	col/o	scop/o (examine)	e—noun (instrument) y—noun (process or action)
rectum	rect/o		ic—adjective
		combining form	**suffix**
anus and rectum	proct/o		
		pleg/a (paralysis)	ia—noun ic—adjective
glands of digestion liver pancreas	hepat/o pancreat/o		

113

answer column
_____

stomat/o

The word root—combining form for mouth is

_____ / _____.

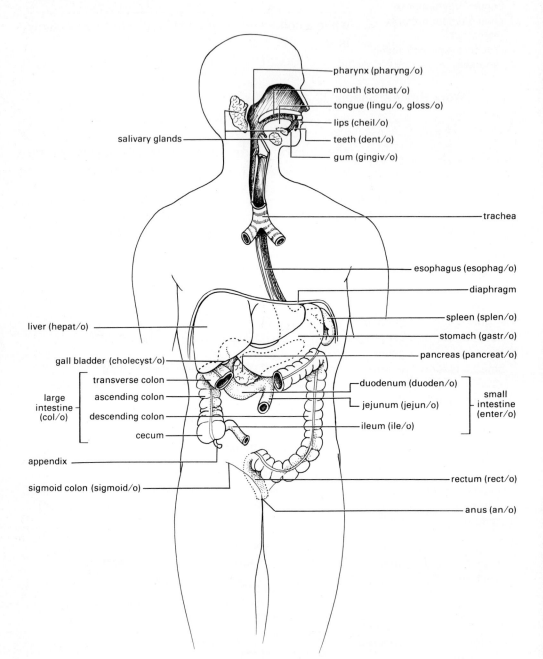

pharynx (pharyng/o)

mouth (stomat/o)

tongue (lingu/o, gloss/o)

lips (cheil/o)

teeth (dent/o)

gum (gingiv/o)

salivary glands

trachea

esophagus (esophag/o)

diaphragm

spleen (splen/o)

liver (hepat/o)

stomach (gastr/o)

pancreas (pancreat/o)

gall bladder (cholecyst/o)

transverse colon

ascending colon

large intestine (col/o)

descending colon

cecum

duodenum (duoden/o)

jejunum (jejun/o)

small intestine (enter/o)

ileum (ile/o)

appendix

rectum (rect/o)

sigmoid colon (sigmoid/o)

anus (an/o)

The digestive system

answer column

inflammation of the
mouth
surgical repair of the
mouth

stomat/algia
stō mə tal′ jē ə

stomat/orrhagia
stō mə tō rā′ jē ə

stomat/o/myc/osis
stō mə tō mī kō′ sis

stomat/o/path/y
stō mə top′ ə thē

stomat/o/scop/e
stō′ mət ə skōp

stomat/o/scop/y
stō mə tos′ kə pē

gloss/o

inflammation of the
tongue

excision of the tongue

712

Stomat/itis means
    ** _____ .

Stomat/o/plast/y means
    ** _____ .

713

Using the word root for mouth, form a word mean-ing:

pain in the mouth

___stomat / dynei a___;

hemorrhage of the mouth

___stomat / orrhagia___.

714

Using the combining form for mouth, build a word meaning:

condition of mouth fungus

stomat / o / myc / osis___;

any disease of the mouth

stomat / o path / y .

715

A micr/o/scop/e is an instrument for examining something small. An instrument for examining the mouth is a

___stomat / o / scop / e___. The

process of examining with this instrument is

___stomat / o / scop / y___.

716

The word root–combining form for tongue is

gloss /o .

Gloss/itis means
    ** _____ .

Gloss/ectomy means
    ** _____ .

717

Using the word root, build a word meaning:

pain in the tongue

gloss / algia ;

pertaining to the tongue

gloss / al .

718

One of the cranial nerves is the hypo/gloss/al. It supplies nerve impulses *_____

_____. A medication which is administered under the tongue is

hypo / gloss / al medication.

719

Using the combining form for tongue, build a word meaning:

prolapse of the tongue

gloss / o / ptosis ;

examination of the tongue

gloss / o / scop / y .

720

Using the information needed from page 107 build a word meaning:

paralysis of the tongue

gloss / o / pleg / ia ;
                    noun

paralysis of the tongue

_____ / / _____ / _____ .
                    adjective

721

Cheil/itis means
          **_____.

Cheil/o/plast/y means
          **_____.

722

The word root for lip is _Cheil_. The combining form for lip is _Cheil / o_ .

116

answer column	
cheil/otomy kī lot′ ə mē	
cheil/osis kī lō′ sis	

723
Build a word meaning:
  incision of the lips

____cheil__ / __otomy____ ;

  condition or disorder of the lips

____cheil__ __osis____ .

---

cheil/o/stomat/o/plast/y
cheilostomatoplasty
kī lō stō mat′ ə plas tē

724
A word meaning plastic surgery of the lips and mouth is

____cheil__ / __o__ / __stomat__ / __o__ / __plast__ / __y____ .

  lip   mouth   repair   suffix .

---

pertaining to the gums

gingiv/o

725
Gingiv/al means
  **_____ .

The word root–combining form for gums is

____gingiv__ / __o____ .

---

gingiv/itis
jin ji vī′ tis
gingiv/algia
jin ji val′ jē ə

726
Build a word meaning:
  inflammation of the gums

____gingiv__ / __itis____ ;

  gum pain ____gingiv__ / __algia____ .

---

gingiv/ectomy
gingivectomy
jin ji vek′ tə mē

gingiv/o/gloss/itis
(You pronounce it.)

727
Build a word meaning:
  excision of gum tissue

____gingiv__ / __ectomy____ ;

  inflammation of the gums and tongue

____gingiv__ / __o__ / __gloss__ / __itis____ .

---

stomach hemorrhage

inflammation of the
  stomach

pertaining to the stomach

728
Gastr/orrhagia means
  **____stom. hemm.____ .

Gastr/itis means
  **____stom. inf.____ .

Gastr/ic means
**____stom. pert.____ .

117

answer column

gastr/ectasia gas trek tā′ zhə	**729** Form a word meaning: dilatation (stretching) of the stomach _gastr / ectasia_; prolapse of the stomach and small intestine _gastro / enter / o / ptosis_.
gastr/o/enter/o/ptosis gas′ trō en tər op tō′ sis	
gastr/o/enter/ic gas′ trō en ter′ ik	**730** Form a word meaning: pertaining to the stomach and small intestine _gastro / enter / ic_; hemorrhage of the small intestine _enter / orrhagia_.
enter/orrhagia en tə rō rā′ jē ə	
enter/o/cele en′ tə rō sēl enter/o/clysis enteroclysis en tə rok′ lə sis	**731** Build a word meaning: intestinal hernia _enter / o / cele_; washing or irrigation of the small intestine _enter / o / clysis_.
enter/o/pleg/ia en tə rō plē′ jē ə	**732** Build a word meaning: paralysis of the small intestine _enter / o / pleg / ia_; dilatation of the small intestine _enter / ectasia_.
enter/ectasia en tə rek tā′ zhə	
prolapse of the small intestine surgical puncture of the small intestine	**733** Enter/o/ptosis means **_prolapse of_ Enter/o/centesis means **_puncture o_
,pertaining to the colon or large intestine surgical puncture of the colon	**734** Col/ic means **_pert. colon_. Col/o/centesis means **_punct. of colon_

118

col/o/pex/y
colopexy
kō′ lō pek sē,
kol′ ō pek sē
col/ostomy
colostomy
ko los′ tə mē

735

Build a word meaning:
  surgical fixation of the colon

___col / o / pex / y___;

  making a new opening into the colon

___col / o / stomy___.

---

col/o/clysis
kō lok′ lə sis

col/o/ptosis
kō lop tō′ sis

736

Build a word meaning:
  washing or irrigation of the colon

___col / o / clysis___;

  prolapse of the colon

___col / o / ptosis___.

---

enter/o

col/o

enter/o/scop/e
en′ tə rō skōp

737

The combining form for small intestine is

___enter / o___.

The combining form for large intestine (colon) is

___col / o___.

An instrument to examine the small intestine is the

___enter / o / scop / e___.

---

rect/o

pertaining to the rectum

a rectal hernia or hernia
 of the rectum

738

The word root—combining form for rectum is

___rect / o___.

Rect/al means
** ___pertaing to___ .

A rect/o/cele is
** ___hern, rectum___.

---

rect/o/clysis
rek tok′ lə sis

rect/o/scop/e
rek′ tə skōp

739

Build a word meaning:
  washing or irrigation of the rectum

___rect / o / clysis___;

  instrument for examining the rectum

___rect / o / scop / e___.

---

rect/o/scop/y
rek tos′ kə pē

740

The process of examining the rectum with a rectoscope is called

___rect / o / scop / y___.

119

answer column	
rectoscopic rek tə skop′ ik	In doing this, the physician has performed a _rect /o/ scop /ic_ adjective examination.

741

Build a word meaning:
   plastic surgery of the rectum

rectoplasty
rek′ tə plas tē

rect /o/ plast /y;

   suturing (stitching) of the rectum

rect/orrhaphy
rek tôr′ ə fē

rectorraphy.

742

Build a word meaning:
   pertaining to the rectum and urethra

rect/o/urethr/al
rek tō yoo rē′ thrəl

rect /o/ urethr /al;

   incision of the bladder through the rectum

rect/o/cyst/otomy
rek tō sis tot′ ə mē

rect /o/ cyst /otomy.

rectum   bladder   incision   .

743

specializes in diseases
  of anus and rectum

A proct/o/log/ist is one who ** _____ .

study of diseases of
  anus and rectum

Proct/o/log/y is
** _____ .

744

Build a word meaning:
   washing or irrigation of anus and rectum

proct/o/clysis
prok tok′ lə sis

proct /o/ clysis;

   paralysis of the opening from the anus

proct/o/pleg/ia or
proctoparalysis

_____ / _____ / _____ / _____ .

745

proct/o/scop/e
prok′ tə skōp

A proctologist examines the rectum with a
proct /o/ scop /e. This

proct/o/scop/y
prok tos′ kə pē

examination is called
proct /o/ scop /y.

120

answer column	

746

Build a word meaning:

suturing of the rectum and anus

proct/orrhaphy
prok tôr′ ə fē

____proct / orraphy____ ;

proct/o/pex/y
prok′ tō pek sē
or
rect/o/pex/y

surgical fixation of the rectum

____rect / o / pex / y____

747

Hepat/ic means
**

_Liver cond.____ .

pertaining to the liver

Hepatomegaly means
**

enlarged liver .

enlargement of the liver

748

Build a word meaning:

inspection (examination) of the liver

hepat/o/scop/y
hep ə tos′ kə pē

____hepat / o / scop / y____ ;

hepat/o/path/y
hep ə top′ ə thē

any disease of the liver

____hepat / o / path / y____ .

749

Build a word meaning:

incision into the liver

hepat/otomy
hep ə tot′ ə mē

____hepat / otomy____ ;

hepat/ectomy
hep ə tek′ t mē

excision of (part of) the liver

____hepat / ectomy____

750

Pancreat/ic means
**

_pancreas____ .

pertaining to the
pancreas

Pancreat/o/lys/is means ** _dest.

destruction of pancreatic
tissue

_____ .

751

Build a word meaning:

a stone or calculus in the pancreas

pancreat/o/lith
pan krē at′ ō lith

____pancreat / o / lith____ ;

pancreat/o/path/y
pan′ krē ə top′ ə thē

any pancreatic disease

____pancreat / o / path / y____ .

121

answer column

pancreat/ectomy
pan' krē ə tek' tə mē

pancreatotomy
pan' krē ə tot' ə mē

752
Build a word meaning:

excision of part or all of the pancreas

pancreat / ectomy ;

incision into the pancreas

_____ / __o tomy_ .

hepatoscopy

hepatorrhaphy

753
Build a word meaning:

examination of liver _hematoscopy_ ;

suture of liver _hematorrhaphy_ .

hepatocele

hepatodynia (algia)

hepatolith

754
Build a word meaning:

hernia of the liver _hematocele_ ;

pain in the liver _hematodynia_ ;

stone in the liver _hematolith_ .

See "Case Study: Operative Report."

splen/ectomy
spli nek' tə mē

splen/o/megal/y

splen/o/ptosis
(You pronounce)

755
splen/o is used in words about the spleen. Build a word meaning:

excision of the spleen

splen / ectomy ;

enlargement of the spleen

splen/o/megal/o ;

prolapse of the spleen

splen/o/ptosis .

splen/o/pex/y

splen/o/path/y

splen/orrhaphy

splen/orrhagia

756
Build a word meaning:

surgical fixation of the spleen

splen/o/pex/y ;

any disease of the spleen

_____ /o/ path/y_ ;

suture of the spleen

_____ / orrhaphy_ ;

hemorrhage from the spleen

_____ /o/rrhagia_ .

122

answer column	
	757
	The spleen is one of the blood-forming organs. Splen/algia means
pain in the spleen	** _____ .
	758
	Splen/ic means
pertaining to the spleen	** _____ .
	759
	Anastomosis is a surgical connection between tubular structures. The word root for esophagus is *esophag/o*. When an entire gastrectomy is performed, a new connection is made between the esophagus and the duodenum. This operation can also be called an
esophag/o/duoden/ ostomy esophagoduodenostomy i sof′ ə gō dōō ə də nos′ tə mē	_____ / ___ / _____ .

123

Fun, wasn't it?

760
Analyze (make your own diagonal divisions):
gastroenterocolostomy

_____

esophagogastrostomy

_____

enterocholecystostomy

_____

Amazing what can be
done with a few odd
word roots!

761
Analyze (make your own diagonal divisions):
jejunoileostomy

_____

duodenocholecystostomy

_____

esophagogastroscopy

_____

Work Review Sheets 14 and 15.

762
Arteries (arteri/o) are vessels (angi/o) that carry
blood from the heart. Veins are vessels that carry
heart · blood back to the _____.

763
A word root–combining form for vein is **phleb/o.**
arteries · Arteriosclerosis is hardening of the _____.
phleb/o/scler/osis · Hardening of veins is called
phlebosclerosis
fleb ō sklə rō′ sis · *phleb/o/scler/osis*

764
Build a word meaning:
excision of a vein
phleb/ectomy · *phleb/ectomy*;
fli bek′ tə mē
fixation of a vein
phleb/o/pex/y · *phleb/o/pex/y*.
fleb′ ō pek sē

765
Build a word meaning:
venous dilatation (stretching)
phlebectasia · *phleb/ectasia*;
fleb ek tā′ zhə

124

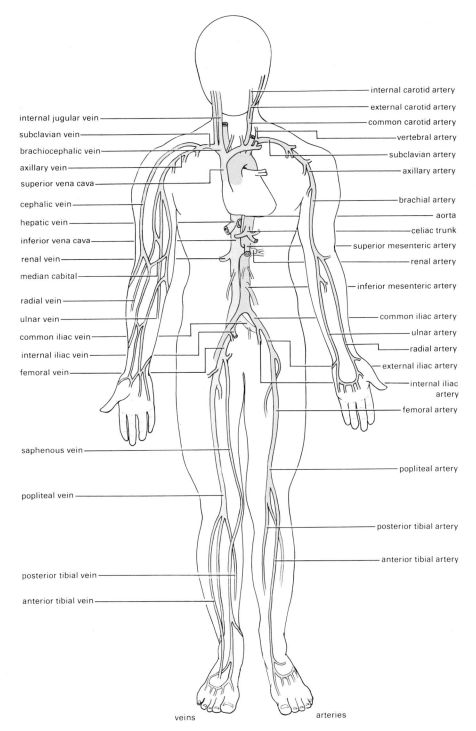

internal jugular vein

subclavian vein

brachiocephalic vein

axillary vein

superior vena cava

cephalic vein

hepatic vein

inferior vena cava

renal vein

median cabital

radial vein

ulnar vein

common iliac vein

internal iliac vein

femoral vein

saphenous vein

popliteal vein

posterior tibial vein

anterior tibial vein

internal carotid artery

external carotid artery

common carotid artery

vertebral artery

subclavian artery

axillary artery

brachial artery

aorta

celiac trunk

superior mesenteric artery

renal artery

inferior mesenteric artery

common iliac artery

ulnar artery

radial artery

external iliac artery

internal iliac artery

femoral artery

popliteal artery

posterior tibial artery

anterior tibial artery

veins

arteries

Veins and arteries

125

answer column
arteriectasia
är tir′ ē ek tā′ zhə
angiectasia
an′ jē ek tā′ zhə

arterial dilatation

____arteri / ectasia____ ;

vessel dilatation

____angi / ectasia____ .

___

766

Phleb/o/plasty means

** ____vein surg. repair____ .

Phleb/otomy means

** ____incision____ .

surgical repair of a vein
  incision into a vein or
  venisection

___

767

Another combining form that you can use as a suffix is **orrhexis.** orrhexis means rupture. Hyster/orrhexis means ** ____uterus rupture____

_____ .

rupture of the uterus

___

768

With orrhexis you learn the last of the ''rrh'' forms. None of the four is a real suffix. But you are fortunate to be able to use them as _____ .

suffixes

___

769

Cyst/orrhexis means

** ____bladder____ .

Enter/orrhexis means

** ____small int.____ .

rupture of the bladder

rupture of the small
  intestine

___

770

Build a word meaning:
  rupture of the heart

____cardi / orrhexis____ ;

  rupture of a vessel

____angio / orrhexis____ .

cardi/orrhexis
kär de ō rek′ sis

angi/orrhexis
an je ō rek′ sis

___

771

Build a word meaning:
  rupture of an artery

____arteri / orrhexis____ ;

  rupture of a vein

____phleb / orrhexis____ .

arteri/orrhexis
är tir ē ō rek′ sis

phleb/orrhexis
fleb ə rek′ sis

126

answer column	

rupture of the tissues of the uterus

metr/orrhexis
mēt rōr ek′ sis

metr / orrhexis

773

Build a word meaning:
   rupture of the liver

hepat/orrhexis

hepat / orrhexis ;

   suturing of the liver

hepat/orrhaphy

hepat / orrhaphy ;

   flowing from the liver

hepat/orrhea
(You pronounce)

hepat / orrhea .

774

Build a word meaning:
   rupture of the bladder

cyst/orrhexis

cyst / orrhexis ;

   hemorrhage from the bladder

cyst/orrhagia

cyst / orrhagia ;

   flowing from the bladder

cyst/orrhea

cyst / orrhea ;

   suturing of the bladder

cyst/orrhaphy
(You pronounce)

cyst / orrhaphy .

775

Esthesia is a word meaning feeling or sensation. **an**
is a form of the prefix **a**. an means

without

_____ .

776

Esthesia means _feeling_ .
   **

feeling or sensation

Analyze the following words:
   esthesiometer

esthesi/o/meter

_____ / ___ / _____

   esthesioscopy

esthesi/o/scop/y

_____ / ___ / ___ / _____

   anesthesia

an/esthesi/a

___ / _____ / ___

   anesthesiology

an/esthesi/o/log/y
(You pronounce)

___ / _____ / ___ / ___ / _____

127

777

Think of the meaning as you analyze the following words:

dysesthesia

_____/_____/_____

dys/esthesi/a

hypoesthesia

_____/_____/_____

hypo/esthesi/a
(You pronounce)

778

Algesia is a noun meaning oversensitivity to pain. Hyper/esthesi/a is a synonym for algesia. Algesia means ** _____

oversensitivity to pain
or hyperesthesia

_____.

779

Analyze the following words (remember to **think** as you analyze):

algesimeter

_____/_____/_____

alges/i/meter

algesic (adjective)

_____/_____

alges/ic

algesia (noun)

_____/_____

alges/ia

analgesia

_____/_____/_____

an/alges/ia
(You pronounce)

780

Analyze the following words (you do the dividing):

analgesia _____

an/alges/ia

hyperalgesia

_____

hyper/alges/ia

paralgesia

_____

par/alges/ia

paralgia

_____

par/algia
(You pronounce)

781

par/a means beside, beyond, near, or abnormal. Paranephritis means

** _____.

inflammation near the
kidney

Parahepatitis means

** _____.

inflammation near the
liver

128

782
Analyze the following words:
  paranephritis

par/a/nephr/itis

_____ / _____ / _____ / _____
  paraplegia

par/a/pleg/ia

_____ / _____ / _____ / _____
  paralysis

par/a/lys/is
(You pronounce)

_____ / _____ / _____ / _____

783
Analyze the following words (you divide them):
  parasalpingitis

par/a/salping/itis

_____
  parahepatitis

par/a/hepat/itis
par/a/oste/o/arthr/o/
  path/y
(You pronounce)

_____
  paraosteoarthropathy

_____

784
Analyze the following words (**phas/o** means speech):
  paraphasia

par/a/phas/ia

_____ / _____ / _____ / _____
  aphasia

a/phas/ia

_____ / _____ / _____
  tachyphasia

tach/y/phas/ia

_____ / _____ / _____ / _____
  bradyphasia

brad/y/phas/ia
(You pronounce)

_____ / _____ / _____ / _____

785
Analyze the following words:
  dysphasia

dys/phas/ia

_____
  hyperphasia

hyper/phas/ia

_____
  dysphonia

dys/phon/ia
hypo/phon/ia
(You pronounce)

_____
  hypophonia

_____

129

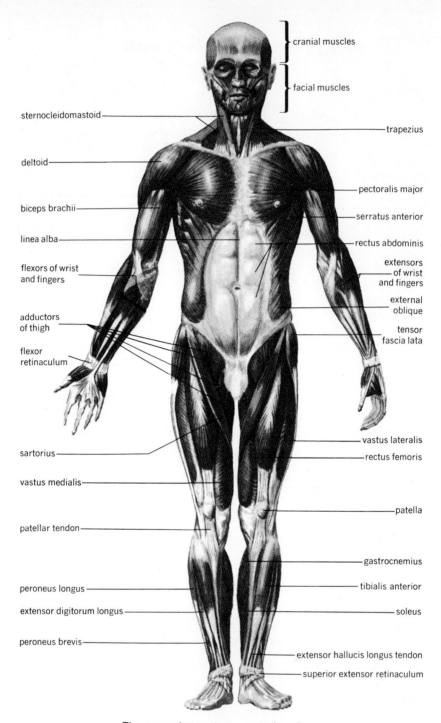

cranial muscles

facial muscles

sternocleidomastoid

trapezius

deltoid

pectoralis major

biceps brachii

serratus anterior

linea alba

rectus abdominis

flexors of wrist
and fingers

extensors
of wrist
and fingers

adductors
of thigh

external
oblique

flexor
retinaculum

tensor
fascia lata

sartorius

vastus lateralis

rectus femoris

vastus medialis

patella

patellar tendon

gastrocnemius

peroneus longus

tibialis anterior

extensor digitorum longus

soleus

peroneus brevis

extensor hallucis longus tendon

superior extensor retinaculum

The muscular system—anterior view

130

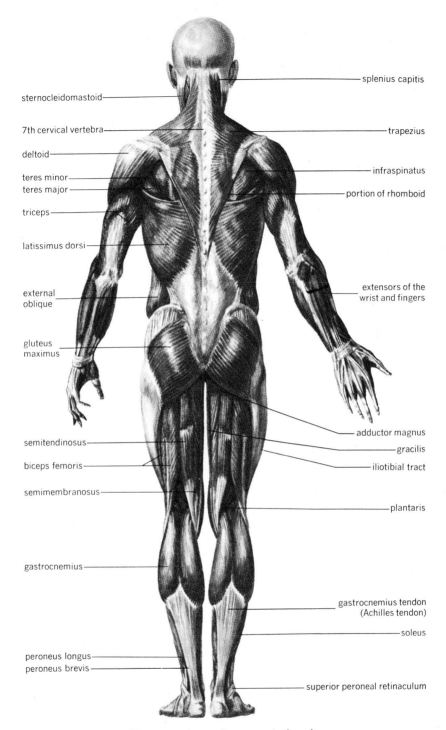

splenius capitis

sternocleidomastoid

7th cervical vertebra

deltoid

teres minor
teres major

triceps

latissimus dorsi

external
oblique

gluteus
maximus

semitendinosus

biceps femoris

semimembranosus

gastrocnemius

peroneus longus
peroneus brevis

trapezius

infraspinatus

portion of rhomboid

extensors of the
wrist and fingers

adductor magnus

gracilis

iliotibial tract

plantaris

gastrocnemius tendon
(Achilles tendon)

soleus

superior peroneal retinaculum

The muscular system—posterior view

131

answer column	

786

phas/o means speech.
phon/o means voice or sound.

rapid speech

Tachyphasia means
** _____.

weak voice (poor etc.)

Dysphonia means
** _____.

787

slow speech

Bradyphasia means
** _____.

absence of voice

Aphonia means
** _____.

pertaining to the voice

Phonic means
** _____.

an instrument for
  measuring intensity
  of voice

A phonometer is
** _____.

788

Analyze the following words:
  phonocardiography

phon/o/cardi/o/graph/y

_____ / _____ / _____ / _____ / _____

  phonomyography

phon/o/my/o/graph/y

_____ / _____ / _____ / _____ / _____

  phonomyogram

phon/o/my/o/gram

_____ / _____ / _____ / _____

  phonology

phon/o/log/y
(You pronounce)

_____ / _____ / _____

789

Myocarditis means inflammation of the heart muscle. My/o is used in words referring to the

muscles

_____.

790

Using the words myogram, myograph, and myography, fill the blanks.

myogram

_____myogram_____ the chart

myograph

_____myograph_____ the instrument

myography

_____myography_____ the process

132

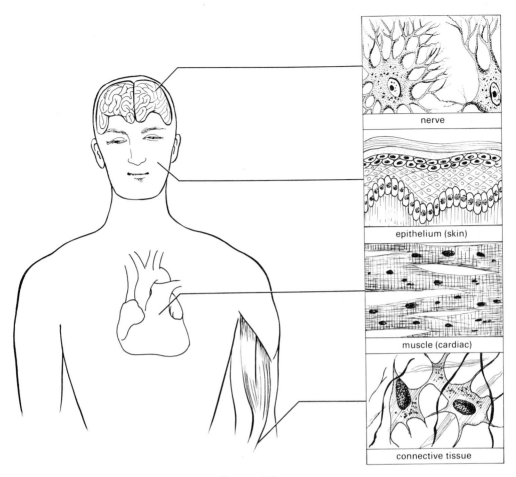

nerve

epithelium (skin)

muscle (cardiac)

connective tissue

Types of tissue

answer column	791
	Analyze (you divide):
my/asthen/ia	myasthenia _____
my/o/brad/ia	myobradia _____
my/o/card/ium	myocardium _____
my/o/card/itis	myocarditis _____
	792
	Analyze:
my/o/fibr/oma	myofibroma _____
my/o/fibr/osis	myofibrosis _____
my/o/fibr/o/sitis	myofibrositis _____

793

If you feel insecure about **myo** words, analyze and check your definitions of:

my/oid

myoid ___resembling___

my/o/lip/oma

myolipoma ___muscle tumor___

my/o/path/y

myopathy ___muscle disease___

794

For your own interest, count how many words you know beginning with my/o. Write the number here. _____ .

over 60

795

When you see my/o, you will think of _____ .

muscles

796

kinesi/o is used in words to mean movement or motion. Brad/y/kinesi/a means ** _____ ___slow___ .

slowness of movement

797

Kinesi/algia means ** ___movement___ .

pain on movement or movement pain

798

Kinesi/algia occurs when you have to move any sore or injured part of the body. Moving a broken arm causes

kinesi/algia
kinesialgia
ki nē sē al' jē ə

_____ .

799

After one's first ride on horseback, almost any movement causes

kinesialgia

_____ .

800

kinesi/ology
kinesiology
ki nē sē ol' ə jē

ology is used like a suffix to mean **study of.** (Remember **ologist?**) The study of muscular movements is _____ / _____ .

134

answer column	
	801 Kinesi/ology is the study of movement. The study of muscular movement during exercise would be done in the field of
kinesiology	_____.
	802 The whole science of how the body moves is embraced in the field of
kinesiology	_____.
abnormally slow movement	**803** Brad/y/kinesi/a means ** _____ .

Work Review Sheets 16 and 17 in Appendix A.

heart double double	**804** **dipl/o** means double. Dipl/o/cardi/a means having a double _____heart_____. Dipl/o/genesis means production of __2__ parts or __2__ substances.
dipl/opia diplopia dip lō′ pē ə	**805** **opia** is an involved form that we can use as a suffix. **opia** means vision. Build a word meaning double vision. ____dipl / opia____.
diplopia	**806** There are many kinds of diplopia. "Crossed eyes" cause one kind of _____.
diplopia	**807** Whenever both eyes fail to record the same image on the brain, ____diplopia____ occurs.
both	**808** **amb/i** means both or both sides. Amb/i/later/al means pertaining to ____both____ sides.
both	**809** An amb/i/dextr/ous person can work well with ____both____ hands.

135

answer column	

810

A word that means both eyes form separate images (vision) is _amb/i/opia_

amb/i/opia
ambiopia
am bē ō' pē

811

The result of separate vision from both eyes is a double image or double vision. Medically, double vision can be expressed either as

_____/_____ or

_____/___/_____ .

dipl/opia

amb/i/opia

812

Look up ambivalence in any dictionary. Read its meaning. Analyze it, and the two words following:

_____/___/_____/_____

_____/___/_____/_____

_____/___/_____/_____

amb/i/valen/ce
am biv' ə ləns
amb/i/valen/cy
am biv' ə lən sē
amb/i/valen/t
am biv' ə lənt

813

A dipl/o/bacteri/um is a bacterium that occurs in pairs or doubly. A coccus that grows in pairs is a

_____/___/_____/_____ .

dipl/o/cocc/us
diplococcus
dip lō kok' əs

814

Hyperopia means farsightedness (vision). A word that means blue vision is

_____/_____ .

cyan/opia
sī ə nō' pē ə

815

neur/o is used in words that refer to nerves. Neur/algia means pain along the course of a

_____ .

nerve

816

Neuroarthropathy is a disease of _____ and _____ .

nerves
joints

817

Neurology is the medical specialty that deals with the nervous system. One who specializes in diseases of the nervous system is a

_____/___/_____/_____ .

neur/o/log/ist
neurologist
noo rol' ə jist

136

neur/itis
noo rī′ tis

neur/o/lys/is
noo rol′ ə sis

neur/o/plast/y
noor′ ə plas tē

818

Build a word meaning:
inflammation of a nerve

_____/_____;

destruction of nerve tissue

neur / o / lys / is;

surgical repair of nerves

neur / o / plast / y.

819

Neur/o/trips/y means surgical crushing of a nerve.
The word root for crushing (usually by rubbing or
grinding) is _____.

trips

820

Trips/is, from which we get **trips/y,** is a Greek word
that means "rub" or "massage." Tripsis can be
carried to the point of crushing or grinding. Surgical
crushing of a nerve is

neur/o/trips/y
noor′ ə trip sē

neur / o / trips / y.

821

In some cases of lithiasis, it may be necessary to
crush calculi so they may be passed. A word to
mean surgical crushing of stones is

lith/o/trips/y

lith / o / trips / y.

822

Look up myel/itis in your dictionary (dictionary work
through Frame 824). From the definition, you con-
clude that **myel** is the word root for

spinal cord
bone marrow

* spine _____ and

* bone marrow _____.

---

myel/o/blast
mī′ ə lō blast
myel/o

823

Find the word myeloblast. Analyze it.

_____/_____/_____

The combining form of myel is _____/_____.

137

answer column	

Find a word meaning:
  pertaining to myelocytes

myel/o/cyt/ic
mī ə lō sit′ ik

_____ / ____ / _____ / ____ ;

herniation of the spinal cord

myel/o/cele
mī′ ə lō sēl

_____ / ____ / _____ ;

defective (poor or bad) formation of the spinal cord

myel/o/dys/plas/ia
mī ə lō dis plā′ zhə

_____ / ____ / dys / plas / ia .

(handwritten margin note: Dysplasia Abnormal formation)

825

plas/ia, plas/is means formation or change in the sense of molding. This kind of formation occurs naturally instead of being done by a plastic surgeon. Dys/plas/ia means ** _____

defective (poor or abnormal) formation

_____ .

826

A/plas/ia means failure of an organ to develop properly. A word that means overgrowth or too much development is

hyper/plas/ia
hyperplasia
hī pər plā′ zhə

_____ / _____ / _____ .

827

If overdevelopment is hyperplasia, underdevelopment is expressed as

hypo/plas/ia
hī pō plā′ zhə

_____ / _____ / _____ .

828

Using myel/o/dys/plas/ia as a model, build a word meaning:
  defective development of cartilage

chondr/o/dys/plas/ia

chondr/o/ dys/ plas/ ia ;

defective formation of bone and cartilage

oste/o/chondr/o/dys/
  plas/ia

oste/ /chondr/o/ dys/ plas/ ia .

829

Form a word meaning inflammation of nerves and spinal cord.

neur/o/myel/itis
neuromyelitis
noor′ ō mī ə lī′ tis

neur /o/ myel/ itis

830

psych/o comes from the Greek "psyche." Both terms mean soul or mind. In a Webster's Collegiate Dictionary, look up psycho and psyche. Read the definitions. Look at how many words in everyday English begin with the word root psych.

---

answer column

free frame

831

Analyze and, using your dictionary, read the meanings of:

psych/o/analysis   psychoanalysis _____

psych/o/surgery   psychosurgery _____

psych/o/somatic   psychosomatic _____

832

Psychiatry is the field of medicine that studies and deals with mental and neurotic disorders. The physician who specializes in this field of medicine is called a

psychiatrist
si kī′ ə trist   _____.

The treatment of mental disorders by a psychiatrist is called

psychotherapy   _____.

833

Psych/o/log/y is the science that studies the mind and mental process. The scientist who works in this field is called a

psych/o/log/ist
psychologist   _____ / ___ / _____ / _____.
sī kol′ ə jist

(Psychiatry is the medical branch of psychology.)

834

Psych/o/genesis means the formation of mental characteristics. A severe mental condition marked by loss of contact with reality, delusions, or hallu-

psych/osis
psychosis   cinations is _____ / _____.
sī kō′ sis

835

Psychoneurosis, an emotional and behavioral disorder is manifest by anxiety. A psych/o/neur/o/tic

psych/o/neur/osis   person is one who suffers from a
psychoneurosis
sī kō noo rō′ sis   _____ / ___ / _____ / _____.

139

836

The patient suffering from a psychoneurosis knows the real from the unreal and only exaggerates reality. Individuals who will not touch others because they fear contact with germs may suffer from

_____ .

psychoneurosis

837

Psychoneuroses (plural) take many forms. Hysteria, psych/asthenia, and neur/asthenia are forms of

_____ .

psychoneuroses

838

In your dictionary read about the **psychopath** and the **psychopathic** personality. Also read the definition of **psychopathy.** In the next frame analyze these three words.

free frame

839

_____

_____

_____

psych/o/path

psych/o/path/ic

psych/o/path/y

sī kop′ ə thē

840

Let your eye wander down the columns of ''psych'' words. Read about any that interest you. Note the information following the words psychiatric and psychoanalysis. All psych/o words refer to

_____ .

mind or soul

841

pharmac/o means drugs or medicine. Neuropharmacology is the study of drugs that affect the nerves. The study of drugs that act on the mind and emotions is _____ / ___ / _____ / _____ .

psych/o/pharmac/o/logy

psychopharmacology

sī kō färm a kol′ a jē

842

In Webster's dictionary look at the words beginning with gnos. They come from the Greek word meaning _____ .

knowledge

843

The words **gnosia** and **gnosis** are medical words built from the Greek word meaning _Knowledge_

_____.

844

Following some dictionary definitions there is a section headed **prog.** This stands for pro/gnos/is, which means foreknowledge or predicting the outcome of a disease. The prefix that means "before or in front of" is _____.

pro

845

Leukemia is a serious disease associated with leukocytes. The _____ for acute leukemia is grave.

prognosis
prog nō' sis

846

Procephalic means **in the front** of the head. Analyze procephalic.

_____ / _____ / _____

Prognostic means giving an indication concerning the outcome of a disease. Analyze prognostic.

_____ / _____ / _____

pro/cephal/ic
prō sə fal' ik

pro/gnos/tic
prog nos' tik

847

di/a means through. Di/ag/nos/is literally means
** _____ .

knowing through
or know through

848

A di/a/gnos/is of a disease is made by studying **through** its symptoms. When a patient tells of having chills, hot spells, and a runny nose, the physician may make a

_____ / ___ / _____ / ____ of a head cold.

di/a/gnos/is
diagnosis
dī əg nō' sis

849

Dialysis is the separation of substances in a solution. Hemodialysis removes waste from the blood by using an artificial kidney.

141

850

The literal meaning of di/a/rrhea is ** _____

_____ .

flowing through

851

Di/a/therm/y means generating heat through (tissues).

di/a means _____ .

therm means _____ .

y is a noun _____ .

through

heat

suffix or ending

852

Dialysis is a process of destroying waste products in the blood by diffusion **through** a membrane. People with kidney failure may need _____ to remove waste products from their blood.

dia/lys/is
dialysis
dī al' i sis

Work Review Sheets 18 and 19.

853

therm/o is the word root-combining form that means heat. An instrument to measure heat is a

_____ / _____ / _____ .

therm/o/meter
thûr mom' ə tər

854

Build a word meaning:

pertaining to heat _____ / _____ ;

oversensitivity to heat

_____ / _____ / _____ ;

formation of (body) heat

_____ / _____ / _____ .

therm/al or therm/ic

therm/o/esthesia or
therm/o/algesia

therm/o/genesis
(You pronounce)

855

Build a word meaning:

abnormal fear of heat

_____ / _____ / _____ / _____ ;

heatstroke (paralysis)

_____ / _____ / _____ / _____ ;

heating through tissue

_____ / _____ / _____ / _____ .

therm/o/phob/ia

therm/o/pleg/ia

di/a/therm/y
(You pronounce)

142

856

If you ever want information about temperature scales or variations of body temperature, you would look in the dictionary for words beginning with

_____ .

therm or therm/o
(Try it!)

857

A micr/o/scop/e is an instrument for examining something small. An instrument for examining "through" is a

_____ / ____ / _____ / _____ .

di/a/scop/e
dī′ ə skōp

858

A diascope is placed on the skin, and the skin is looked at "through" the instrument to see superficial surface lesions, etc. The word part for (through)

is ____ / ____ .

di/a

859

micr/o/ means small. Hydr/o/cephal/us is a condition involving fluid in the head. An abnormally small head is

_____ / ____ / _____ / _____ .

micr/o/cephal/us
mī krō sef′ ə ləs

860

Microcephalus limits the size of the brain. Most microcephalic people are mentally retarded. Occasionally a baby is born with an unusually small head or

_____ / ____ / _____ / _____ .

micr/o/cephal/us

861

A cyst is a sac containing fluid. You also use cyst/o in building words pertaining to cysts.

A very small cyst is a

_____ / ____ / ____ .

micr/o/cyst
mī′ krō sist

A very small cell is a

_____ / ____ / ____ .

micr/o/cyt/e
mī′ krō sīt

A small heart is

_____ / ____ / _____ / _____ .

micr/o/cardi/a
mī krō kär′ dē ə

143

microsurgery
mī krō sûr′ jər ē

large

macr/o/cyt/e(s)
mak′ rō sīt(s)

macr/o/cephal/us

macr/o/blast

macr/o/cocc/us
(You pronounce)

abnormally:
   large tongue
   large ear(s)
   large nose
   large lips

dactyl

dactyl/o

862

Surgery performed on minute structures, using a microscope and small instruments, is

_____.

863

macr/o is the opposite of micr/o. Macr/o is used in words to mean _____.

864

Things that are macr/o/scop/ic can be seen with the naked eye. Very large cells are called

_____ / _____ / _____ / _____.

865

An abnormally large head is

_____ / _____ / _____ / _____.

A large embryonic (germ) cell is a

_____ / _____ / _____.

A very large coccus is called a

_____ / _____ / _____ / _____.

866

Macr/o/gloss/ia means ** _____.
Macr/ot/ia means ** _____.
Macr/o/rhin/ia means ** _____.
Macr/o/cheil/ia means ** _____.

867

Macr/o/dactyl/ia means abnormally large fingers or toes. The word root for fingers or toes is

_____.

868

Another way of saying large fingers or toes is dactyl/o/megal/y. The combining form for finger or toe is _____ / ____.

869

A finger or toe is called a digit. (When you see digit, finger, or toe, use dactyl/o.) Build a word meaning:

dactyl/itis
dak ti lī′ tis

dactyl/o/spasm
dak′ ti lō spaz əm

dactyl/o/gram
dak til′ ə gram

inflammation of a digit

_____ / _____ ;

cramp or spasm of a digit

_____ / _____ / _____ ;

a fingerprint

_____ / _____ / gram .

870

Macr/o/dactyl/ia means

abnormally large
 fingers and toes
 (digits)

** _____ .

Poly/dactyl/ism means too many

fingers or toes
 (digits)

** _____ .

871

(pol/y) is a combining form that means too many or too much. Pol/y/ur/ia means excessive amount of urine. When a person drinks too much water,

pol/y/ur/ia
pol i yoor′ ē ə

_____ / _____ / _____ / _____ results.

872

Pol/y/neur/o/path/y means disease of many nerves. The word for inflammation of many nerves is

pol/y/neur/itis
polyneuritis
pol ē noo rī′ tis

_____ / _____ / _____ / _____ .

873

Build a word meaning:
  inflammation of many joints

pol/y/arthr/itis
pol ē är thrī′ tis

_____ / _____ / _____ / _____ ;

pol/y/neur/algia
pol ē noo ral′ jē ə

  pain in many nerves

_____ / _____ / _____ / _____ ;

pol/y/ot/ia
pol ē ō′ shē ə

  state of having too many or more than two ears

_____ / _____ / _____ / _____ .

874

having many cysts

Pol/y/cyst/ic means ** _____ .

eating too much

Pol/y/phag/ia means ** _____ .

excessive fear of things
(too many phobias)

Pol/y/phob/ia means ** _____ .

145

875

Syn/dactyl/ism means a joining of two or more digits. The prefix that means together or joined is

_____ .

syn

together or joined

876

Syn/ergetic means working together. Drugs that work together to increase each other's effects are

called _____ / _____ drugs.

syn/ergetic
synergetic
sin ər jet′ ik

877

Synergetic muscles are muscles that work together. There are three muscles that work together to flex the forearm. They are _____

muscles.

synergetic

work together

878

APC tablets are frequently more effective for killing pain than aspirin alone. This is because aspirin, phenacetin, and caffeine are _____ drugs.

synergetic

879

Analyze synarthrosis:

prefix _____

word root (joint) _____

condition _____

syn

arthr

osis

880

A syn/arthr/osis is an immovable joint. The joining bones are fused together. When bones are fused at a joint so that there is no movement, the joint is a

_____ / _____ / _____ .

syn/arthr/osis
synarthrosis
sin är thrō′ sis

881

drom/o comes from the Greek word for "run." A drom/o/mania is an insane impulse to wander or roam. You usually use **drom** with the prefixes syn and pro. In this usage, it is a symptom that is "running."

146

882

A syn/drome is a variety of symptoms occurring (running along) together. The complete picture of a disease is its

_____.

883

Look up syndrome in your dictionary. Read about Korsakoff's syndrome. Note some others. A syndrome due to alcoholism is

_____

_____.

884

Expectant mothers are warned not to drink alcohol during pregnancy to prevent deformities in the newborn, known as fetal alcohol _____.

885

Behavior changes and hyperemesis following a viral infection are symptoms occurring together that may indicate Reye's _____.

886

Pro/drome means running before (a disease). Symptoms that indicate an approaching disease are its _____ / _____.

887

The sneezes that come before a common cold are the _____ of the cold.

888

Pro/drom/al is the adjectival form of pro/drom/e. A rash that shows before the true macules of measles is called a _____ / _____ / _____ rash.

pro/drom/al
prodromal
prod' rə məl, prō drō' məl

889

Chicken pox has a rash that precedes macules, or a _____ rash.

Work Review Sheets 20 and 21.

147

answer column

890

Pol/y/dips/ia means excessive thirst (desire for **too much** fluid). The word root for thirst is

_____.

dips

891

Pol/y/dips/ia can be caused by something as simple as eating too much salt. A highly salted meal may cause

_____ / / _____ / _____.

pol/y/dips/ia
polydipsia
pol i dip′ sē ə

892

Polydipsia can be caused by something as complex as an upset in pituitary secretion. If the pituitary gland secretes too much of one hormone, salt is retained in the body, and

_____ results.

polydipsia

893

Large doses of some forms of cortisone also cause

_____.

polydipsia

894

Dips/o/mania is a way of saying alcoholism. A person who drinks excessively of alcoholic beverages suffers from

_____ / / _____.

dips/o/mania
dipsomania
dip sō mā′ nē ə

895

A dips/o/mani/ac is a person who suffers from dips/o/mania. A person with Korsakoff's syndrome is usually a

_____ / / _____ / _____.

dips/o/mani/ac
dipsomaniac
dip sō mā′ nē ak

896

Build a word meaning:
   condition of thirst

_____ / _____;

   treatment by (limiting) water intake

_____ / / _____ / _____.

dips/osis
dipsosis
dip sō′ sis
dips/o/therap/y
dip sō ther′ ə pē

148

Use these ideas to help you through Frame 921.

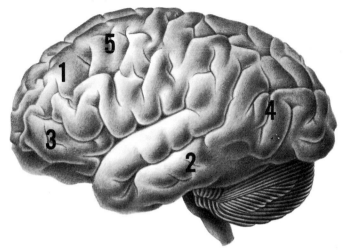

In the biologic sciences there are many directional words. This page is to help you understand the use of nine of them. Label the drawings on the basis of the information given. Use this page while working Frames 897–921.

DIRECTIONAL WORD	COMBINING FORM	MEANING
dorsal	dors/al–dors/o (back)	near or on the back
ventral	ventr/al–ventr/o (belly)	near or on the belly side of the body
anterior	anter/ior–anter/o (before)	toward the front or in front of
posterior	poster/ior–poster/o (behind after)	following or located behind
cephalic	cephal/ic–cephal/o (head)	upward–toward the head
caudal, caudad	caud/al–caud/o (tail)	downward–toward the tail
medial	medi/al–medi/o (middle)	toward the midline
lateral	later/al–later/o (side)	toward the side–away from the midline

Dog

897 _____

898 _____ 902 _____

899 _____ 901 _____

900 _____

Human

903 _____

904 _____ 908 _____

905 _____ 907 _____

906 _____

Check your answers with the correct labels at the bottom of the next page.

Analyze the words in the next four frames.

answer column

anter/o/lateral

anter/o/medi/al

anter/o/superior
(You pronounce)

909

anterolateral _____
(side)
anteromedial _____
(middle)
anterosuperior _____
(above)

poster/o/later/al

poster/o/extern/al

poster/o/intern/al
(You pronounce)

910

posterolateral _____
(side)
posteroexternal _____
(outer)
posterointernal _____
(inner)

anter/o/poster/ior

dors/o/cephal/ad

dors/o/dynia
(You pronounce)

911

anteroposterior _____

dorsocephalad _____

dorsodynia _____

ventr/ad

ventr/otomy

ventr/o/scop/y
(You pronounce)

912

ventrad _____

ventrotomy _____

ventroscopy _____

Dog

dorsal

anterior   posterior

cephalic   caudad
                al
ventral

Human

cephalic

ventral   dorsal

anterior   posterior

caudad
al

150

913

To find a word root for the **navel,** look up navel in the dictionary (see illustration on page 61). A synonym for navel is _____.

914

The combining form for umbilicus is **omphal/o.** Inflammation of the umbilicus is

_____.

915

Turn to words beginning with omphal. The combining form for omphal is _____ / ____.

916

Words beginning with omphal/o refer to the

_____.

917

Using omphal/o, build a word meaning:
  pertaining to the navel

_____ / _____;

  excision of the umbilicus

_____ / _____;

  herniation of the navel

_____ / ____ / _____.

omphal/ic
om fal' ik

omphal/ectomy
om fə lek' tə mē

omphal/o/cele
om' f ə lō sēl
om fal' ō sēl

918

Build a word meaning:
  umbilical hemorrhage

_____ / _____;

  discharge flowing from the navel

_____ / _____;

  rupture of the navel

_____ / _____.

919

Words containing omphal/o refer to the _____,
which is also called the

_____.

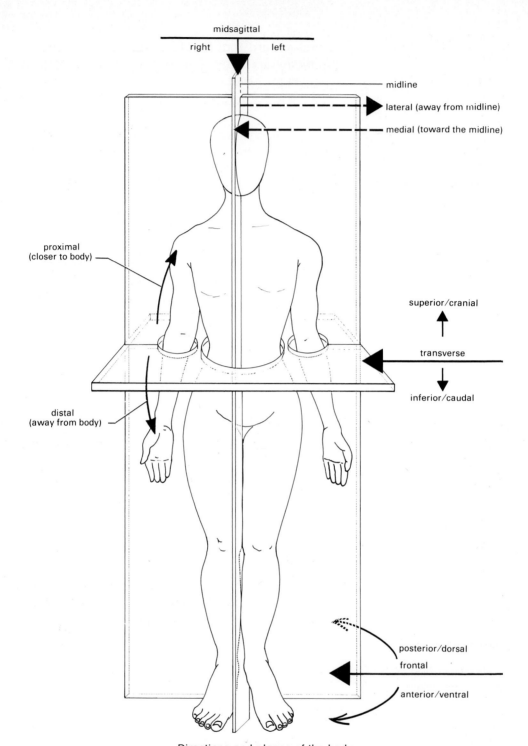

Directions and planes of the body

cephal/ad

cephal/o/trips/y

cephal/o/meter

toward tail

caud/a

caud/ate

caud/ation
(You pronounce)

air

aer/o/phob/ia
air ō fō′ bē ə

aer/o/therap/y

aer/o/cele
(You pronounce)

bi/o/log/y

living things or life

living things

920
cephalad _____

cephalotripsy _____

cephalometer _____

921
cauda _____

caudate _____

caudation _____

922
aer/o is used in words to mean air. You undoubtedly know the words aer/ial, and aer/ialist. You probably use an aer/o/sol bomb to kill insects. Aer/o always makes you think of _____.

923
Using what you need of aer/o, build a word meaning:

abnormal fear of air

_____ / _____ / _____ ;

treatment with air

_____ / _____ / _____ .

herniation containing air

_____ / _____ .

924
bios is the Greek word for life. Bi/o/chemistry is the study of chemical changes in living things. The science (study of) living things is

_____ / _____ / _____ .

925
A biologist is one who studies
**
_____ .

Biogenesis is the formation of
**
_____ .

153

answer column	
	926
	An an/aer/o/bi/c plant or animal cannot live in the presence of air (**an**—without). Analyze anaerobic:
an	prefix (without) _____
aer/o	combing form (air) _____ / ____
bi	word root (life) _____
c	adjectival ending ____
	927
aer/o/bi/c	If anaerobic means existing without air (oxygen), build a word that means needing air (oxygen) to live (adjectival form):
aerobic	
air ō′ bik	_____ / __ / _____ / ____ .
	928
	Use aerobic or anaerobic in the following sentences (four frames).
	The bacterium that causes pneumonia requires air to live. These bacteria are considered
aerobic	_____ bacteria.
	929
	The tetanus bacillus causes lockjaw. Lockjaw can develop only in closed wounds where air does not penetrate (e.g., stepping on an old nail). The tetanus bacillus is an _____ bacterium.
anaerobic	
an ə rō′ bik	
	930
	Botulism is a serious type of food poisoning. It occurs from eating improperly canned meats and vegetables. Cans do not admit air. The bacillus that causes botulism is _____ .
anaerobic	
	931
	A physician who opens a wound so the air can reach it is protecting against infection by an _____ bacterium.
anaerobic	
	932
living or live	A biopsy is an examination of
	_____ tissue.

154

933

A combining form that means color is chrom/o. The Greek word for a color is "chroma." There are English words chroma and chrome. Chrom/o makes you think of _____.

color

934

A chromocyte is any colored cell. An **embryonic** color (pigment) cell is called a

_____ / _____ / _____.

chrom/o/blast
chromoblast
krō' mō blast

935

Build a word meaning:
   destruction of color (in a cell)

_____ / _____ / _____ ;

chrom/o/lys/is
krō mol' ə sis

   formation of pigment (color)

_____ / _____ / _____ ;

chrom/o/genes/is
krō mō jen' ə sis

   instrument for measuring amount of color in a substance

_____ / _____.

chrom/o/meter
krō mom' ə tər

936

A chrom/o/phil/ic cell is one that takes a stain easily. Some leukocytes stain deeper than others. They are more

_____ / _____ / _____ than

the less easily stained leukocytes.

chrom/o/phil/ic
chromophilic
krō mō fil' ik

937

Some cells will not stain at all. They are not

_____.

chromophilic

938

Some cells stain with one dye but not with another. They are differentially

_____.

chromophilic

939

Chromophilic means
** _____. The

staining easily

155

answer column

a/chrom/o/phil/ic
achromophilic
ā krō mō fil′ ik

word that means something does not (without) stain easily is

_____/_____ /____/_____/_____.

bad, painful, or
  difficult

well or easy

940

dys means * _____.
The opposite of **dys** is **eu. eu** means
                                              **
                                                _____.

eu/peps/ia
yōō pep′ sē ə
eu/pept/ic
yōō pep′ tik
eu/pne/a
yōōp nē′ ə

941

Form the word that means the opposite of:

  dys/peps/ia _____/_____/_____ ;

  dys/pept/ic _____/_____/_____ ;

  dys/pne/a _____/_____/_____ .

942

Form the opposite of:
  dys/kinesi/a

  _____/_____/_____ ;

  dys/esthesi/a

  _____/_____/_____ ;

  dys/phor/ia

  _____/_____/_____ .

eu/kinesi/a
yōō ki nē′ zhə

eu/esthesi/a
yōō es thē′ zhə

eu/phor/ia
yōō fôr′ ē ə

943

Dys/tocia means difficult labor. Eutocia means
**_____.

                                                              Test 4

easy or normal labor
  and childbirth

think

944

If you work a frame and have forgotten what the word root means, **look it up** in your medical dictionary. You may also find it in the review sheets in Appendix A.

945

thanatos is a Greek word meaning death. The combining form for death is **than/o.** When someone has an easy or peaceful death, it is called
_____/_____/_____. Many ethical medical questions surround the subject of
_____.

eu/than/asia
euthanasia
yoo than a′ zhə

euthanasia

156

946

Another area of ethical importance is the study of **eu/gen/ics.** Researchers are working on ways of improving the human race through genetic engineering. Look up **eugenic** in your dictionary and analyze the word parts.

good

eu _____

form or produce

gen _____

adjective ending

ic _____

947

Recall that **enter/o** is the combining form for small intestine. Infections of the small intestine can be viral, bacterial, or parasitic and cause pain and diarrhea. This painful or difficult small intestinal condition is called _____/_____.

dys/entery
dysentery
dis′ en tair e

948

Travelers are cautioned not to drink water in countries with poor sanitation systems to avoid contracting amebic _____.

dysentery

949

men/o is used in words referring to the menses. Men/ses is another way of saying men/struation. **men/o** in any word should make you think of _____.

menses or menstruation

950

Men/o/pause means permanent cessation of

_____.

Men/orrhagia means

** _____.

menstruation or menses

excessive menstruation
 or menstrual
 hemorrhage

951

Men/arche refers to a girl's first menstrual period. Build a word meaning:
 flow of menses

_____/_____;

painful (bad or difficult) menstrual flow

_____/_____/_____

men/orrhea
men ə rē′ ə

dys/men/orrhea
dis men ə rē′ ə

157

952
Build a word meaning:
absence (without) menstrual flow

_____ / _____ / _____ ;

stopping of menstrual flow

_____ / ___ / _____ .

953
Stasis means the act or condition of stopping or controlling. Hem/o/stasis means
**
_____ .

A word meaning control of flow in veins is

_____ / ___ / _____ .

phleb/o/stasis
fli bos′ tə sis
or ven/o/stasis

954
Build a word meaning:
control of flow in arteries

_____ / ___ / _____ ;

control of lymph flow

_____ / ___ / _____ .

955
Syphilis is a venereal disease. Read about the disease in your dictionary. Note the origin of the word. Look at the words beginning with **syphil.** The combining form used in words referring to this disease is _____ / ___ .

956
Analyze the last four words in your dictionary that begin with syphil.

_____

_____

_____

_____

syphil/o/psych/osis
syphil/osis
syphil/ous
syphil/o/phobe
syphil/o/phob/ia
syphil/o/phyma
syphil/o/tropic
syphil/o/therap/y

(The answers will vary with the dictionary used. Pick the proper four in the answer column.)

158

answer column	

957
Build a word meaning:
a syphilitic tumor

syphiloma

_____ / _____ ;

resembling syphilis

syphiloid

_____ / _____ ;

syphilopathy
(You pronounce)

any syphilitic disease

_____ / _____ / _____ / _____ .

958
pseud/o means false. A pseudocyesis is a false pregnancy. A pseudoscience is a

false science

  * _____ .

959
Pseud/o/mania is a psychosis in which patients falsely accuse themselves of crimes. Pseud/o/paralysis means ** _____

false paralysis
(paralysis not due to
nerve damage)

_____ .

960
Build a word meaning:
a false cyst

pseud/o/cyst
sōō′ dō sist

_____ / _____ / _____ ;

false edema

pseud/o/edema
sōō dō i dē′ mə

_____ / _____ / _____ ;

false or imaginary sensation

pseud/o/esthesi/a
sōō dō es thē′ zhə

_____ / _____ / _____ / _____ .

Look up and learn the meaning of **edema.**

961
Build a word meaning:
false hypertrophy

_____ / _____ / _____ / _____ ;

pseud/o/hyper/troph/y

false tuberculosis

_____ / _____ / _____ / _____ ;

pseud/o/tubercul/osis

false

pseud/o/syphil/is
(You pronounce)

_____ / _____ / _____ / _____ .

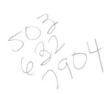

159

962

The viscera are the internal organs of the body. Viscerad means toward the viscera. Viscerogenic is also a word. The word root–combining form for viscera is _____ / ____.

viscer/o

963

In the words viscer/o/motor, viscer/o/pariet/al, and viscer/o/pleur/al, viscer/o refers to

_____.

organs
(internal organs)

964

Build a word meaning:
  prolapse of organs

_____ / ____ / ____ ;

viscer/o/ptosis
vis ər op tō′ sis

  pain in organs

_____ / ____ ;

viscer/algia
vis ər al′ jē ə

  pertaining to organs

_____ / ____ .

viscer/al
vis′ ər əl

965

Analyze:
  viscerosensory

_____

viscer/o/sens/ory

visceroskeletal

_____

viscer/o/skelet/al

viscerogenic

_____

viscer/o/gen/ic

Work Review Sheets 22 and 23.

966

lapar/o means abdominal wall. A laparectomy is an excision of part of the

* _____.

abdominal wall

967

Process of examining the abdominal cavity with a scope is called

_____ / ____ / ____ .

lapar/o/scopy
laparoscopy
lap ə ròs′ kō pē

968

An incision into the abdominal wall is a

_____/_____.

A suturing of the abdominal wall is

_____/_____.

969

Analyze the following words:

    laparohepatotomy _____

    laparocolostomy _____

    laparogastrotomy _____

970

There may be longer words than this. If there are, there are not many. Analyze it for fun. Think of the word parts.

Laparohysterosalpingo-oophorectomy _____

971

pyr/o is used in words to mean heat or fever. (Remember the funeral pyres on which the early Greeks and Romans burned their dead?) A pyromaniac is one who has a madness for starting or seeing

_____.

972

Pyr/exia means fever. A condition of heat (heartburn) is _____/_____.

973

Build a word meaning:

    instrument for measuring heat

_____/_____/_____;

    destruction by fever

_____/_____/_____;

    abormal fear of fire

_____/_____/_____/_____.

answer column

answer column	
fever or high body temperature, etc.	**974** A pyr/o/toxin is a toxin (poison) produced by ** _____.
sweat	**975** Hydr/o means water or fluid. Hidr/o means sweat. A hidr/o/cyst/oma is a cystic tumor of a _____ gland.
inflammation of sweat glands	**976** Hidr/o/aden/itis means ** _____ _____.

hidr/osis
 	
 hyper/hidr/osis
 	
 hidr/orrhea
 (You pronounce)
	977
	 There are three words that mean excessive sweating. Analyze them:
	    hidrosis
	    _____
	
	   hyperhidrosis
	    _____
	
	   hidrorrhea
	    _____

absence of sweat	**978** The word an/hidr/osis means ** _____ _____.
water or fluid sweat	**979** Both hydr/o and hidr/o are pronounced alike. Hydro with a "**y**" means _____. Hidro with an "**i**" means _____.
glyc/o/gen glycogen glī′ kō jen	**980** **glyc/o** comes from the Greek word for "sweet." Glyc/o/gen is "animal starch" formed from simple sugars. The cells of the body use a simple sugar, glucose, to release energy. To use its reserve fuel supply of animal starch, the body must convert _____ / _____ / _____ to glucose.
	981 Glucose is used by the muscles to release energy. Glycogen is the reserve food supply of glucose.

162

answer column	
glycogen	Glucose is the usable form from the reserve supply of _____.

982

Glycogen is potential sugar. Glucose is usable sugar. In words, glyc/o should make you think of

sugar or sweet _____ .

983

Glyc/emia means sugar in the blood. Hyper/glyc/emia means

too much sugar in the
blood (high blood sugar)   ** _____ .

984

Hyper/glyc/emia means high blood sugar. The word that means low blood sugar is

hypoglycemia
hī pō glī sē′ mē ə   _____ .

985

The formation of glycogen from food is

glyc/o
glycogenesis
glī kō jen′ ə sis   _____ / ____ / ____ .

986

The breakdown (destruction) of sugar is

glyc/o/lys/is
glī kol′ ə sis   _____ / ____ / _____ / ____ . The

discharge (flow) of sugar from the body is

glyc/orrhea
glī kō rē′ ə   _____ / ____ .

987

sugar
fat   Glyc/o/lip/id should make you think of two foods: _____ and _____ .

Work Review Sheets 24 and 25.
The following chart is for use in building words through Frame 1014.

COMBINING FORM OF LOCATION		MEANING
	ect/o	outer–outside
	end/o	inner–inside
	mes/o	middle
	retr/o	backward–behind
	par/a	near

163

988

The blast/o/derm is an embryonic disk of cells that gives rise to the three main layers of tissue in humans. The outer germ layer is called the ect/o/derm. The inner germ layer is called the

_____ / ___ / _____ .

end/o/derm
endoderm
en' dō dûrm

989

Between the ectoderm and endoderm is a middle germ layer called the

_____ / ___ / _____ .

mes/o/derm
mesoderm
mez' ō dûrm

990

The ectoderm forms the skin. The nervous system arises from the same layer as the skin. This layer is the _____ .

ectoderm
ek' tō dûrm

991

Sense organs and some glands are also formed from the _____ .

ectoderm

992

The end/o/derm forms organs inside the body. The stomach and small intestine arise from the

_____ .

endoderm

993

The lungs are also formed by the inner layer of tissue, or the _____ .

endoderm

994

The mesoderm forms the organs that arise between the ectoderm and endoderm. Muscles are formed by the _____ .

mesoderm

995

Bones and cartilages also arise from the middle layer of tissue, or the _____ .

mesoderm

The blastoderm gives rise to the three germ layers. They are:

answer column

outer _____ ;

middle _____ ;

inner _____ .

ectoderm

mesoderm

endoderm

997

The ectoderm, mesoderm, and endoderm form everything that is in the body.

ect/o means _outer_ .

end/o means _inner_ .

mes/o means _middle_ .

outer

inner

middle

998

Something produced within an organism is said to be end/o/genous. Something produced outside an organism is

_____ / _____ / _____ .

ect/o/genous
ectogenous
ek toj′ ə nəs

999

Ect/o/cyt/ic is an adjective meaning outside a cell. An adjective meaning inside a bladder is

_____ / _____ / _____ / _____ .

end/o/cyst/ic
endocystic
en dō sis′ tik

1000

Prot/o/plasm is the substance of life. The protoplasm that forms the outer limit of the cell is called

_____ / _____ / _____ . The protoplasm

within the cell is called

_____ / _____ / _____ .

ect/o/plasm

end/o/plasm
(You pronounce)

1001

End/o/crani/al is an adjective meaning within the cranium. An adjective meaning within cartilage is

_____ / _____ / _____ / _____ .

end/o/chondr/al
en dō kon′ drəl

1002

End/o/enter/itis means inflammation of the lining of the small intestine. Build a word meaning:

    pertaining to the lining of the heart (adjective)

_____ / _____ / _____ ;

endocardial or
  endocardiac

inflammation of the lining of the colon

_____ / __ / _____ / _____ .

Note the involved development of the word ectopic (out of place):

ect/o — outside

top/os — place (Greek word)

ic — adjectival suffix

1003

ectopic
ek top' ik

An ectopic pregnancy occurs outside of the uterus. A heart on the right side of the body is an

_____ heart.

1004

ectopic

If endometrium occurs in the fallopian tubes, a fertilized egg can lodge in it, thus causing pregnancy. This is an _____ pregnancy.

1005

ectopic

An embryo's development in the abdominal cavity is also an _____ pregnancy.

1006

mes/o/neur/itis

mes/o/col/ic

mes/o/cephal/ic

mes/o/cardi/a

Think of the meaning while you analyze:

mesoneuritis _____

mesocolic _____

mesocephalic _____

mesocardia _____

1007

retr/o/col/ic
ret rō kol' ik

Build an adjective meaning:

behind the colon

_____ / __ / _____ / _____ ;

behind the mammary (gland)

retr/o/mammary
ret rō mam' ə rē
retr/o/stern/al
ret rō stûr' nəl

_____ / __ / mammary ;

behind the stern/um

_____ / __ / _____ / al .

1008

Ante/version means turning forward. The word for turning backward is

_____ / ___ / _____ .

1009

The retr/o/periton/eum is the space _____ the peritoneum. An inflammation of this space is called

_____ / ___ / _____ / _____ .

1010

Ant/e/flexion means forward bending. Retr/o/ flexion means ** _____

_____

1011

Par/a/centr/al means

** _____ .

Par/a-/appendic/itis means ** _____

_____ .

1012

Build a word meaning:

inflammation around the bladder

_____ / ___ / _____ / _____ ;

inflammation of tissues around the vagina

_____ / ___ / _____ / _____ .

1013

Build a word meaning inflammation of tissues:

around the liver   _____ ;

around the kidney   _____ .

1014

ect/o means ___ outer ___ .

end/o means ___ inner ___ .

mes/o means ___ middle ___ .

par/a means ___ around ___ .

retr/o means ___ behind ___ .

167

1015

aut/o is a word root–combining form that means self. You already recognize **auto** in such ordinary English words as aut/o/mobile (a self-propelled vehicle) and aut/o/bi/o/graph/y. Aut/o means

_____.

self

1016

Immunity is the body's protection from many diseases. If a person's **own** body produces antibodies to its **own** tissues, _____ has occurred.

auto/immun/ity
autoimmunity
ô tō im ū′ ni tē

1017

Acquired immune deficiency syndrome (AIDS) is characterized by a lack of **immunity.** Previously healthy people who develop AIDS may not be able to fight off diseases.

1018

Aut/o/di/a/gnos/is means diagnosing one's own diseases. Aut/o/derm/ic pertains to dermoplasty with

** _____.

one's own skin

1019

Aut/o/nom/ic means self-controlling. Aut/o/lys/is means

** _____.

self-destruction or
self-destroying

1020

Aut/o/phag/ia means biting one's self. A word that means abnormal fear of being alone is

_____ / _____ / _____.

aut/o/phob/ia
autophobia
ô tō fō′ bē ə

1021

In the blanks provided, analyze the following:

autohemotherapy _____

autopsychosis _____

autoplasty _____

aut/o/hem/o/therap/y
aut/o/psych/osis
aut/o/plast/y
(You pronounce)

168

When you analyze a word, think of its meaning. If you have forgotten a part of the word, look it up.
Analyze:

answer column		
aut/o/phob/ia	autophobia	_____
aut/o/phag/ia	autophagia	_____
aut/o/nephr/ectomy	autonephrectomy	_____
(You pronounce)		

Learn to count with prefixes.

PREFIX	MEANING	PREFIX	MEANING
mono	one	quint	five
multi	many	sex	six
nulli	none	septa	seven
primi	first	octa	eight
uni	one	nona	nine
bi (diplo)	two	deca	ten
tri	three	centa	one hundred
quad	four	kilo	one thousand

---

answer column

1023

mon/o means one or single. You know it in the ordinary English words monotony, monopoly, and monogamy. Whenever you see mon/o, you think of

one

_____ .

1024

A mon/o/graph deals with a single subject. A mon/o/nucle/ar cell has _____ nucleus.

one

1025

Mon/o/man/ia is an abnormal preoccupation with one subject only. Build a word meaning:

mon/o/cyt/e

one cell   _____ / _____ / _____ / _____ ;

mon/oma
(You pronounce)

one tumor   _____ / _____ .

1026

Analyze the following words:

mon/o/my/o/pleg/ia
mon/o/neur/al
mon/o/nucle/osis
(You pronounce)

monomyoplegia   _____

mononeural   _____

mononucleosis   _____

169

1027

Mult/i means the opposite of mon/o. Mult/i means

many or more than one

** _____ .

1028

In ordinary English, you are acquainted with multi in the words multiply and multitude. Something composed of multiple parts has _____ parts.

many

1029

Something that is mult/i/capsular has

many capsules

* _____ .

1030

Mult/i/glandular is an adjective meaning

* _____ .

Mult/i/cellular is an adjective meaning

* _____ .

Mult/i/nuclear is an adjective meaning

* _____ .

many glands

many cells

many nuclei

1031

A mult/i/par/a is a woman who has brought forth (borne) more than one child. **Par** is the word root meaning to bear. Mult/i/par/ous is the adjectival form of

_____ / ___ / ___ / ___ .

multi/i/par/a
multipara
mul tip'ə rə

1032

Mult/i/par/a **always** refers to the mother. Mult/i/par/ous may refer to the mother or may mean multiple birth (twins or triplets). When desiring to indicate that a woman has borne more than one child, use the noun

_____ .

multipara

1033

Multiparous is the adjectival form of _____ .
To indicate that twins are born, say

_____ birth.

multipara
multiparous
mul tip' ər əs

1034

To indicate that triplets are born, say

_____ birth. If

multiparous

ten children were born, you would still use the
adjective

multiparous

_____ .

1035

Null/i means none. To nullify something is to bring
it to nothing. There are not many medical words
using null/i; but when you do see it, it means

_____ .

1036

a woman who has never
borne a child

A null/i/par/a is

**

_____ .

prim/i/par/a
prī mip′ ər ə

Prim/i means first. A woman who is having her first
child is a

_____/_____/_____/_____ .
(noun)

1037

Analyze the following and define:

null/i/par/a

nullipara _____
(noun)

null/i/par/ous

nulliparous _____
(adjective)

prim/i/par/a

primipara _____
(noun)

1038

Give the word root–combining form for:

null/i

none _____/_____

mon/o

one (single) _____/_____

mult/i

many _____/_____

par/o

bear _____/_____

prim/i

first _____/_____

Work Review Sheets 26 through 29.

PREFIXES OF PLACE

These prefixes often cause difficulty in word building because of their similarity. The explanations should be helpful. These forms will probably require extra work. This is your first introduction to prefixes of place. Use this information **carefully** while working through Frame 1063.

PREFIX	MEANING	SENSE OF MEANING
ab	from	away from
de	from	down from or from—resulting in less than
ex	from	out from

<table>
<tr><td>answer column</td><td>

1039

You have already learned **ab** as the opposite of **ad. ad** means toward. **ab** means _____.
</td></tr>
<tr><td>from</td><td></td></tr>
</table>

1040

Ab/duct/ion means moving away from the midline. Ab/norm/al means going
* _____ the normal.

answer: away from

1041

Ab/or/al means away from the mouth. Ab/errant means wandering * _____ the normal course.

answer: away from

1042

An ab/irritant is something that takes pain
* _____ the patient. Ab/ lact/ation means taking the baby
* _____ the breast.

answer: away from
answer: away from

1043

Abort was, literally, built by joining the prefix ab, away from, to a word part meaning to be born. When an abortion is performed the fetus is taken * _____ the mother. To abrade the skin is to scrape some of the skin * _____ its surface.

answer: away from
answer: away from

172

answer column	
	1044
	Analyze the words:
ab/duct	abduct _____
ab/neur/al	abneural _____
ab/articulat/ion	abarticulation _____

	1045
from	**de** is another prefix that means _____.

	1046
	One who de/scends the stairs comes down from a
	higher level. A de/scending nerve tract comes
down from	*_____ the brain.

	1047
	A de/scending nerve tract carries descending im-
down from	pulses *_____ the brain.

	1048
	Deciduous leaves fall from a tree. ''Baby teeth''
deciduous	that fall from a child's mouth are called
dē sij′ o͞o əs	_____ teeth.

	1049
	A de/coction is made by boiling down a fluid. While
	a de/coction is boiling down to a thicker substance,
from	water is being taken _____ it.

	1050
	When water is taken from a substance, the sub-
	stance is less than it was. De/hydr/ation takes
from	water _____ something.

	1051
	When water is taken from prunes, de/hydr/ation
de/hydr/ation	occurs. When water is taken from a cell,
dehydration	
dē hī drā′ shən	_____ / _____ / _____ also
	occurs.

	1052
	When something is de/hydr/ated, it is less than
	it was. When water is lost from the body due to
de/hydr/ated	excessive vomiting, the patient is
dē hī′ drā tid	_____ / _____ / _____ .

173

1053

Vomiting can cause dehydration. A high fever can also cause _____.

dehydration

1054

When calcium is removed from the bones, there is less calcium than formerly. This process is called _____/_____.

de/calcification
dē kal′ si fi kā′ shən

1055

Decalcification can occur from many causes. When a pregnant woman does not eat enough calcium for the growing baby, her own bones will be robbed of calcium; and

_____

will occur.

decalcification

1056

Since vitamin D helps control calcium metabolism, inadequate vitamin D in the diet can account for some _____.
Parathyroid imbalance can also cause

_____.

decalcification

decalcification

1057

ex also means from, but in the sense of
* _____.

out from

1058

Ex/eresis means the taking out (from) any part of the body. To excise is to cut _____ and remove a part.

out

1059

To exhale is to breathe out waste matter _____ the body.

from

1060

Ex/cretion is the process of **ex**pelling (or getting out from the body) a substance. Expelling urine is urinary _____.

excretion
(You pronounce)

174

answer column	

1061

Expelling carbon dioxide is called respiratory _____. Expelling sweat is dermal _____ .

excretion
excretion

1062

Expelling menses is menstrual _____ .
Expelling fecal matter is gastrointestinal

_____ .

excretion

excretion

1063

Try to work this summary frame without referring to page 172. Give the prefix meaning **from** in the following sense:

away from   _____

out from   _____

down from or from, resulting in less than

_____

ab

ex

de

1064

narc/o is the word root-combining form for sleep. A narc/o/tic is a drug that produces sleep. Opium produces deep sleep. Opium is a

_____ /   / _____ .

narc/o/tic
narcotic
när kot′ ik

1065

A narcotic produces insensibility as well as sleep. A narcotic should be used only when advised by a physician. Codeine produces sleep. Codeine is a

_____ .

narcotic

1066

Morphine is also a _____ .

narcotic

1067

Since narcotics can also cause addiction, a physician must have a narcotic license in order to dispense or write orders for _____ (plural).

narcotics

1068

The **condition** induced by narcotics is called

_____ / _____ .

narc/osis
narcosis
när kō′ sis

175

narc/o/leps/y narcolepsy när′ kō lep sē	**1069** Narc/o/leps/y means seizure or attacks of sleep. A person who is absolutely unable to stay awake suffers from _____ / __ / _____ / ____
narcolepsy	**1070** Narcolepsy is uncontrollable. A person may fall sound asleep standing at a bus stop. This is _____.
narcolepsy	**1071** A cerebroma, cerebral arteriosclerosis, and paresis are some causes of sleep seizures, which are called _____.
sleep	**1072** **narc/o** any place in a word makes you think of _____.
equal	**1073** **is/o** is used in words to mean equal. Something that is is/o/metr/ic is of _____ dimensions.
equal	**1074** Something that is is/o/cell/ular is composed of _____ cells.
is/o/ton/ic isotonic ī sō ton′ ik	**1075** An is/o/ton/ic solution has the same osmotic pressure as red blood cells. Blood serum is an _____ / __ / _____ / ____ solution.
isotonic	**1076** Intr/a/ven/ous glucose is another _____ solution.
isotonic	**1077** Any solution that will not destroy red blood cells because of pressure difference is an _____ solution.

1078

Build a word meaning:
fingers or toes of equal length

_____ / _____ / _____ / ism _____ ;

pertaining to equal temperature

_____ / _____ / _____ / _____ .

1079

an is a prefix meaning without. Something that is without equality is unequal. The combining form

for unequal is _____ / _____ / _____ .

1080

Anis/o/cor/ia means that the pupils of the eyes are

of _____ size.

1081

Anis/o/mast/ia means that a woman's breasts are

of _____ size.

1082

Anis/o/cyt/osis means that cells are of unequal sizes. This word is commonly limited to red blood cells in medical usage. A word indicating a condi-

anis/o/cyt/osis
anisocytosis
an ī′ sō sī tō′ sis

tion of inequality in cell size is

_____ / _____ / _____ / _____ .

1083

Normal red blood cells are the same size (7.2 microns). An abnormal condition resulting in un-equal size of red blood cells is

_____ .

1084

Red blood cells are formed in the bone marrow. An unhealthy bone marrow can result in unequal red blood cells or

_____ .

1085

Lack of hemoglobin can also cause

_____ .

177

Use the following information to work Frames 1086 through 1105.
This is another group of prefixes of place.

PREFIX	MEANING	DIFFERENTIATION
di/a	through	used with the word root-combining forms for medical terminology
per	through	prefix from Latin: used more often in ordinary English
peri	around	prefix from Greek used with the word root-combining forms for medical terminology
circum	around	Latin prefix used more often in ordinary English

answer column

1086

Peri/articular means around articulations or joints.
Peri/tonsill/ar means

around the tonsil

      *_____.

---

around the colon or
  pertaining to around
  the colon

1087

Peri/col/ic means

      *_____.

---

peri/chondr/al
perichondral
per i kon' dr ə l

1088

Peri/dent/al means around a tooth. A word that
means around a cartilage is

_____ / _____ / _____.

1089

Build a word meaning:
  inflammation around a gland

peri/aden/itis

_____ / _____ / _____;

  inflammation around the vagina

peri/colp/itis

_____ / _____ / _____;

  inflammation around the liver

peri/hepat/itis

_____ / _____ / _____;

  excision of tissue (pericardium) around the heart

peri/cardi/ectomy
(You pronounce)

_____ / _____ / _____.

1090

Another prefix that means around is

circum

_____.

178

1091

Circum/ocular means _____ the eyes.

around

1092

Circum/or/al means _____ the mouth.

around

1093

Circum/scribed means limited in space (as though a line were drawn around it). A hive is limited in space—does not spread. A hive may be called a _____ wheal.

circumscribed
sûr kəm skrīb'd

1094

A boil is also limited in the space it covers. A boil is a _____ lesion.

circumscribed

1095

Pimples and pustules are also

_____ lesions.

circumscribed

1096

Moving toward is ad/duct/ion.
Moving away is ab/duct/ion.
Moving around (circular motion) is

_____ / _____ / _____ .

circum/duct/ion
circumduction
sûr kəm duk' shən

1097

There are two prefixes that mean through. The one that you would expect to use more often in medical terminology is _____ / _____ .

di/a

1098

You have already learned di/a/gnos/is, which means knowing _____, and di/a/therm/y, which means heating

_____ .

through

through

1099

Build a word meaning:
   flowing through (drop the o)

   _____ / / _____ ;

   pertaining to heating through

   _____ / / _____ / _____ .

1100

Per/for/ation (noun) means puncturing

   _____ .

1101

To per/for/ate means to puncture or make a hole

_____ .

1102

The past tense of per/for/ate is per/for/ated. An ulcer that has eaten through the stomach wall has

_____ (past tense)

it.

1103

Ulcers can also _____
(present tense) the duodenum.

1104

When ulcers perforate an organ, a

_____ / _____ / ation   (noun) is formed.

1105

Percussion (noun) means a striking through. Read the section on percussion in a dictionary. Analyze the word here.

   _____ / _____ / _____

1106

Summarize:
Two prefixes meaning through are _____ and
_____ / _____ .

Two prefixes meaning around are
_____ and _____ .

Test 5

	1107
death	**necr/o** is used in words pertaining to death. Necr/o/cyt/osis is cellular _____.
	1108
dead	A necr/o/parasite is one that lives on _____ organic matter.
necr/osis necrosis ne krō′ sis	**1109** Necr/osis refers to a condition in which dead tissue is surrounded with healthy tissue. Certain diseases can cause _____/_____ of the bones.
necrosis	**1110** When blood supply is cut off from an arm, gangrene sets in. This results in _____ (death) of the arm tissue.
necrosis	**1111** When gangrene occurs anywhere in the body, _____ is seen.
	1112 Build a word meaning: excision of dead tissue
necr/ectomy	_____/_____ ;
	incision into (dissection of) a dead body
necr/otomy	_____/_____ ;
necr/o/phob/ia (You pronounce)	abnormal fear of death _____/___/_____/_____ .
necr/o/psy necropsy nek′ rop sē	**1113** There are two ways of saying postmortem (after death) examination. One is aut/o/psy. The other is _____/___/ psy .
necr/o/tic necrotic ne kro′ tik	**1114** Cyanotic is the adjectival form of cyanosis. Build the adjectival form necrosis.

1115

phil/ia is the opposite of phob/ia; **phobia** is abnormal fear of. **philia** is ** _____
attraction to.

abnormal or unusual

1116

Necr/o/phob/ia is an abnormal fear of dead bodies. Necr/o/phil/ia is

* _____ .

abnormal attraction
  to dead bodies

1117

Words that can end in phob/ia, can end in phil/ia. Morbid fear of water is

_____ / ___ / _____ / _____ .

Strong attraction to water is

_____ / ___ / _____ / _____ .

hydro/o/phob/ia

hydr/o/phil/ia
hī drō fil' ē ə

1118

Think of the meaning while building words opposite to:

    hemat/o/phob/ia

_____ / ___ / _____ / _____ ;

    pyr/o/phob/ia

_____ / ___ / _____ / _____ ;

    aer/o/phob/ia

_____ / ___ / _____ / _____ ;

    aut/o/phob/ia

_____ / ___ / _____ / _____ .

hematophilia

pyrophilia

aerophilia

autophilia
(You pronounce)

1119

phil/o is the word root–combining form that means

    ** _____ .

attraction to
liking
loving

1120

Can you think of a nonmedical word that involves phil/o? If so, write it here.

_____

philosopher
philosophy
philology
etc.

Work Review Sheets 30 and 31.

182

1121

hom/o in words means same. Hom/o/genized milk has the same amount of cream throughout. Hom/o/gland/ular means pertaining to the

same gland

*_____.

1122

same

Hom/o/therm/al means having the _____ body temperature.

1123

Hom/o/later/al means pertaining to the

same

_____ side.

1124

Hom/o/sex/ual means being attracted to the same sex. When men are attracted to men much more than to women, they are said to be

hom/o/sex/ual
homosexual
hō mō sek′ shoo əl

_____ / / _____ / _____.

1125

When women are attracted to women rather than to men, they too are called

homosexual

_____.

1126

heter/o is the opposite of hom/o. **heter/o** means

different

**_____.

1127

different

Heter/opia means _____ vision in each eye.

1128

Heter/o/sex/ual means being attracted to a

different

_____ sex.

1129

Look up the meaning of homogeneous and heterogeneous in your dictionary. Understand and know these words.

Analyze them here.

hom/o/gene/ous
hō mō jē′ nē əs
heter/o/gene/ous
het ər ō jē′ nē əs

_____ / / _____ / _____

_____ / / _____ / _____

183

1130

Think of the meaning while you form **opposites** of the following:

hom/o/lys/is

heter/o/lys/is

_____ / _____ / _____ / _____

hom/o/genesis

heter/o/genesis

_____ / _____ / _____

hom/o/sex/ual

heter/o/sex/ual

_____ / _____ / _____ / _____

1131

syn and **sym** are different forms of the same prefix. syn and sym mean _____

together or joined

1132

You have already learned **syn** in the words syndactylism, synergetic, synarthrosis, and syndrome. (Review Frames 875 through 883.)

1133

syn is the form of the prefix that is used to mean fixed or joined, except when it is followed by the sound of **b**, **m**, **f**, **ph**, or **p**. Then _____ is used.

sym

1134

Sympathy is an ordinary word that has a special medical meaning. Read this meaning in your medical dictionary. From either a medical or Webster's dictionary, find what it takes to fill this blank: sym + path/os, the Greek word for

suffering (medical)
feeling (standard)

_____ .

1135

A sym/physis is a growing together of parts. Sym/blephar/on means ** _____

eyelids have grown
 together or adhesions
 of the eyelids

_____ .

1136

Build a word meaning:
  lower extremities are grown together (united)

sympodia

_____ / pod / ia ;

184

excision of a sympathetic nerve

_____ / path / _____;

tumor of a sympathetic nerve

_____ / _____ / _____.

sympathectomy

sympathoma
(You pronounce)

1137
Find a fairly **common** word in your medical dictionary in which **sym** is followed by **m**. (There are only two or three to choose from.) One is
** _____.

symmetry
symmetric
symmetrical

1138
Find a **common** word in your medical dictionary that is used in ordinary English in which **sym** is followed by **b**. It is ** _____.

symbol or symbolism

1139
syn and sym both mean together. **sym** is used when followed by the sound of the letters, __, __, __, __, and _____. syn is used in other medical words.

b m p f ph

1140
super and **supra** are both prefixes that mean above or beyond. Analyze the following words in which super and supra are used. Think of the meaning of the word as you analyze it. If necessary, consult a dictionary.

1141
Super

super/fici/al

super/cili/ary

super/infect/ion

super/ior/ity

super/leth/al

super/numer/ary

superficial	_____
superciliary	_____
superinfection	_____
superiority	_____
superlethal	_____
supernumerary	_____

1142
Supra

supra/lumb/ar

supra/pub/ic

supralumbar	_____
suprapubic	_____

185

supra/crani/al	supracranial _____
supra/ren/al	suprarenal _____
supra/ren/oma	suprarenoma _____
supra/ren/o/path/y	suprarenopathy _____

1143

In a dictionary, look up words beginning with super. Write the number of columns of words beginning with super in the blank indicated below. Do the same with supra.

approximately:
$5\frac{1}{4}$, $\frac{1}{3}$

                                                    super   supra

Webster   _____   _____

---

super is used more frequently in modern English

supra is used more frequently in straight medical words

1144

Draw a conclusion about **super** and **supra** from your answer in the last frame.

super is ** _____.

supra is ** _____.

---

a and **an** are prefixes that mean without.
Examine the following list of words.

an/al/ges/ia	a/bi/o/tic
an/aph/ia	a/blast/em/ic'
an/em/ia	a/chol/ia
an/encephal/us	a/derm/ia
an/esthes/ia	a/febrile
an/iso/cyt/osis	a/galact/ia
an/idr/osis	a/kinesi/a
an/irid/ia	a/lali/a
an/onych/ia	a/men/o/rrhea
an/op/ia	a/pne/a
an/ur/ia	a/reflex/ia
an/ur/esis	a/seps/is

Draw a conclusion.
  Use **a** if it is followed by a

consonant   _____.

vowel   Use **an** if it is followed by a

             _____.

More prefixes! Use this chart to work Frames 1145 through 1168.

PREFIX	MEANING	SPECIAL COMMENT
epi	over–upon	
extra	outside of beyond in addition to	
infra	below–under	almost always below a part of the body almost always adjectival in form There are fewer words beginning with **infra** than with **sub**
sub	under–below	Many words of all kinds begin with sub
meta	beyond–after occurring later in a series	also used with chemical names

answer column

1145

The epi/gastr/ic region is the region

over the stomach

       * _____ .

1146

Epi/splen/itis means inflammation of the tissue

over the spleen

  * _____ .

1147

Build a word meaning:

inflammation of the area over the bladder

epi/cyst/itis
ep i sis tī′ tis

     _____ / _____ / _____ ;

epi/nephr/itis
ep i nef rī′ tis

inflammation (of the tissue) upon the kidney

     _____ / _____ / _____ .

1148

Build a word meaning:

excision of the tissue upon the kidney

epi/nephr/ectomy
ep i nef rek′ tə mē

     _____ / _____ / _____ ;

epi gastr/orrhaphy
ep i gas trôr′ ə fē

suture of the region over the stomach

     _____ / _____ / _____ .

187

epi/derm/al /ic	**1149** Build a word meaning pertaining to (the tissue) upon the skin _____ / _____ / _____ ; (the tissue) covering the cranium _____ / _____ / _____ ;
epicranial	
episternal (You pronounce)	the area above the stern/um _____ / _____ / _____ .

outside of or beyond	**1150** Extra/nuclear means ** _____ the nucleus of a cell.

outside of or beyond	**1151** Extra/uterine means ** _____ the uterus.

extra-/articul/ar eks trə är tik′ yə lər	**1152** Think of the meaning as you analyze: extra-articular (articulation-joint) _____ / _____ / _____
extra/cyst/ic eks trə sis′ tik	extracystic _____ / _____ / _____
extra/dur/al eks trə door′ əl	extradural (dura covers brain) _____ / _____ / _____

extra/genit/al	**1153** Think of the meaning as you analyze: extragenital _____ / _____ / _____
extra/hepat/ic	extrahepatic _____ / _____ / _____
extra/cerebr/al	extracerebral _____ / _____ / _____

adjectives	**1154** Look at the words in the last two frames. Draw a conclusion. **extra** is used as a prefix in words that are usually _____ (nouns/adjectives).

188

below–under	**1155** **infra** is a prefix that means _____.
below or under	**1156** Infra/mammary means _____ the mammary gland.
below or under	**1157** Infra/patell/ar means _____ the patella (kneecap).
under or below	**1158** **sub** is a prefix that means _____.
under below	**1159** Sub/abdominal means _____ the abdomen. Sub/aur/al means _____ the ear.
under or below	**1160** The prefixes infra and sub are sometimes confusing in word building. For that reason, you will build words that can take either prefix. When you see sub or infra, you will think of _____ or _____.
infra/stern/al sub/stern/al supra/stern/al	**1161** Using stern/o, build two words meaning below the sternum. _____ / _____ / al _____ / _____ / A word meaning above the sternum is supra / _____ / _____.
infra/cost/al sub/cost/al supra/cost/al	**1162** Using cost/o, build two words meaning under the ribs. _____ / _____ / _____ / _____ / A word meaning above the ribs is _____ / _____ /.

189

1163

Using pub/o, build two words meaning under the pubis.

_____ / _____ / _____

_____ / _____ / _____

A word meaning above the pubis is

_____ / _____ / _____.

1164

meta is a prefix used in many ways. Look at the chart on page 187 to discover its meanings.

1165

Analyze the term **metaphysics.** It is the study of things

** _____ .

1166

meta/carpal/s
metacarpals
me tə kar′ palz

The bones of the hand that are beyond the carpals (wrist) are the _____ .

1167

meta/tarsal/s
metatarsals
me tə tar′ salz

The bones of the foot that are beyond the tarsals (ankle) are the _____ .

1168

meta/stas/is
metastasis
me tas′ tə sis

A metastasis occurs when a disease spreads beyond its point of origin. A metastatic (adj.) tumor is a secondary growth from a malignant tumor. This secondary growth is a _____ .

1169

You have now learned your prefixes of location. You should review them by making a list of them, with their meaning plus anything special about them.

1170

sepsis is a noun meaning a poisoned state caused by absorption of pathogenic bacteria and their products into the bloodstream. A noun meaning a state without or free from sepsis is

a/seps/is
asepsis
ə sep′ sis, ā sep′ sis

_____ / _____ / _____.

answer column	
a/sept/ic aseptic ə sep' tik, ā sep' tik	**1171** Sept/ic is the adjectival form of sepsis. The adjectival form for the word meaning free from infection is ___/___/___ .
infection with pus in the bloodstream	**1172** Sept/i/cemia is an infection in the bloodstream. Sept/o/py/emia means ** _____ .
sept/o (used most) or seps/o	**1173** Study the last two frames. A word root–combining form for infection is _____/___ .
seps/is sept/ic a/seps/is a/sept/ic	**1174** Review the material from Frames 1170 through 1173. noun for infection _____/_____ adjective for infected _____/_____ noun for a state free from infection ___/___/_____ adjective for free from infection ___/___/_____
against against	**1175** **anti** is a prefix meaning against. An anti/pyretic is an agent that works _____ a fever. An anti/toxin is an agent that works _____ a toxin.[†]
against	**1176** An anti/narcotic is an agent that works _____ narcotics.
against	**1177** An anti/biotic is an agent that works _____ various infections.
anti/rheumatic	**1178** Build an adjective describing the agent that works against: rheumatic disease _____/_____ ;

[†] **Note:** A toxin is a poisonous substance produced by an organism.

191

anti/spastic

anti/toxin
(You pronounce)

spastic disease

_____ / _____ ;

toxins

_____ / _____ .

1179

Build an adjective describing the agent that works against:

convulsive states

anti/convulsive

_____ / _____ ;

arthritic diseases

anti/arthritic

_____ / _____ ;

anti/toxic
(You pronounce)

toxic states

_____ / _____ .

1180

The adjective denoting a drug that works against infection is

antiseptic
an ti sep′ tik

_____ / _____ .

1181

against

contra is a prefix that also means against. contra is usually used with modern English words. To contra/dict someone is to speak _____ what the person is saying.

1182

against

Contra/ry things are _____ each other. A contra/ry person is usually one who is

against

_____ your wishes.

1183

against

In medical terminology, contra is mainly confined in use to four words. However, in these four words contra still means _____ .

1184

Analyze these four words:

contraindication

contra/indicat/ion

_____ / _____

contra/cept/ive

contraceptive

_____ / _____ / _____

contra/volition/al

contravolitional

_____ / _____ / _____

contra/later/al
(You pronounce)

contralateral

_____ / _____ / _____

Don't count it wrong if you miss the second diagonal. (If you get it right, you should feel good.)

1185

Using the words in Frame 1184 fill the following blanks with a word whose literal meaning is:

contravolitional

against volition _____

contraindication

against indication _____

contraceptive

against conception _____

contralateral
(You pronounce)

against the side _____

1186

Using these same words and a medical dictionary, if necessary, fill in the blanks with the word that covers the more extended meaning:

contraceptive

device to prevent conception _____

contralateral

pertaining to the opposite side _____

contravolitional

against the will _____

contraindication
(You pronounce)

symptoms make a particular
treatment inadvisable _____

1187

Using the noun given, build the other parts of the same word:

contra/indicat/e
contra/indicat/ed
(You pronounce)

_____ contra/ / indicat/ / ion _____ (noun)

_____ / _____ / _____ (verb)

1188

trans is a prefix meaning across or over. To trans/

across or over

port a cargo is to carry it _____ the ocean
or land.

193

answer column	
across or over	**1189** Trans/position means literally position _____.
trans/position transposition trans pə zish′ ən	**1190** Transposition means literally placed across. When an organ is placed across to the other side of the body (from where it normally is found) _____/_____. occurs.
transposition	**1191** Cardi/ac transposition means that the heart is on the right side of the body. If the stomach is on the right side of the body, the condition is gastr/ic _____.
transposition	**1192** The liver belongs on the right side of the body. If a patient's liver is on the left side of the body, the condition is hepat/ic _____.

Work Review Sheets 32 and 33.

across or over	**1193** When a trans/fusion is given, blood is passed _____ from one person to another.
trans/sexual trans/illumin/ation trans/vagin/al trans/thorac/ic trans/urethr/al (You pronounce)	**1194** **Analyze:** transsexual _____ transillumination _____ transvaginal _____ transthoracic _____ transurethral _____
	1195 Transpiration is the act of carrying water vapors across lung or skin tissue to eliminate them from the body. Breathing is respiration. Breathing consists of the following two processes: expiration and

ex/pir/ation

in/spir/ation

inspiration

not

not

in/compet/ence
incompetence
in kom′ pə təns

incompetence

incompetence

incompetent

in or not

inspiration. Think of the meaning as you analyze:
expiration

_____/_____/_____

inspiration

_____/_____/_____

1196

Look at the words in Frame 1195. The word that means breathing **in** is

_____.

1197

in is a prefix that means in or not. In/compatible drugs are drugs that do _____ mix with each other.

1198

In/compet/ency occurs in an organ when it is _____ able to perform its function.

1199

In/compet/ence is a noun. When the ile/o/cec/al valve cannot perform its function, the result is ileocecal

_____/_____/_____

1200

When blood seeps back through the aortic valves, call it aortic

_____.

1201

When a person is not able to take care of himself or herself, you may call it ment/al

_____. You may
even say the person is mentally

_____ (adjective).

1202

in is a prefix that means _____ or _____.

195

1203

To in/cis/e is to cut into. This is a verb. The noun
from in/cis/e is _____/_____/_____.

in/cis/ion
incision
in sizh' ən

1204

itis is the suffix for

_____/_____.

1205

Analyze:

  inject   _____

  injected   _____

  injector   _____

  injection _____

in/ject
in/ject/ed
in/ject/or
in/ject/ion
(Do you know the
  meaning?)
(You pronounce)

1206

In Frame 1205 the prefix **in** means _____.

1207

Analyze:

  insane   _____/_____
  insomnia

        _____/_____

  insanitary

        _____/_____

1208

In Frame 1207, the prefix **in** means _____.

1209

Mal is a French word that means bad. **mal** is also
a prefix that means bad or poor. Mal/odor/ous
means having a _____ odor.

1210

Mal/aise means a general feeling or illness or poor
feeling. Mal/form/ation means ** _____
_____.

1211

Mal/nutrition means
_____ .

poor nutrition

Mal/position means
_____ .

bad (abnormal)
position or placement

1212

Before people knew that mosquitoes carry malaria, they thought this disease was caused by bad air. Analyze malaria. _____

mal/aria
malaria
mə lair′ ē ə

1213

Analyze these words involving the disease malaria:

    malarial   _____

mal/ari/al
mal/ari/ous
mal/ari/o/log/y
mal/ari/o/therap/y
(You pronounce)

    malarious   _____

    malariology   _____

    malariotherapy _____

1214

Look at the words in the last two frames. Now find the word root–combining form for the disease malaria. _____ / _____

malari/o

1215

The tri/ceps muscle has _____ heads.
A tri/cusp/id valve has _____ cusps.
The tri/gemin/al nerve has _____ branches.

three
three
three

1216

A bi/cusp/id is a tooth with _____ cusps.
Bi/foc/al glasses have _____ foci in one lens.
A bi/furc/ation has _____ forks or branches.

two
two
two

1217

A uni/corn has _____ horn.
Uni/ov/al pertains to twins who develop from _____ ovum. Uni/vers/al means combined into _____ whole.

one

one
one

answer column	

1218

Later/al means pertaining to the side. Build a word meaning pertaining to:

uni/later/al

    one side

_____ / _____ / _____ ;

bi/later/al

    two sides

_____ / _____ / _____ ;

tri/later/al
(You pronounce)

    three sides

_____ / _____ / _____ .

1219

tri/angle

A tri/later/al figure looks like this △. You call this a _____ / _____ .

1220

Mult/i/cell/ular means made of many cells. Build a word meaning:

    made of two cells

bi/cell/ular

_____ / _____ / _____ ;

    made of one cell only

uni/cell/ular
(You pronounce)

_____ / _____ / _____ .

1221

Some cells are mult/i/nucle/ar in nature. Build a word meaning:

    having one nucle/us

uni/nucle/ar

_____ / _____ / _____ ;

    having two nucle/i

bi/nucle/ar
(You pronounce)

_____ / _____ / _____ .

1222

Mult/i/para refers to a woman who has had more than one child. Build a word meaning:

    a woman who has had one child

uni/para
yoo nip′ ər ə

_____ ;

bi/para
bip′ ər ə

    a woman who has had two children

_____ ;

tri/para
trip′ ər ə

    a woman who has had three children

_____ .

198

1223

To bi/furc/ate is to divide into two forks. When an artery divides into two, it

_____ / _____ / _____ (s) .

bi/furc/ates
bifurcates
bī′ fər kāts

1224

Bifurcate is a verb. The noun is bifurcation. When a nerve divides into two branches, a

_____ (noun) is

formed.

1225

Various ducts in the body also form

_____ (noun–

plural).

1226

uni   means _____ .

bi   means _____ .

tri   means _____ .

Mult/i   means _____ .

PREFIX	MEANING	EXPLANATION
semi	half	Used with modern English words or words closer to modern English
hemi	half	Used more with straight medical words

1227

There are two prefixes that mean half. They are _____ and _____ .

1228

Form a word that means:
   half circle

_____ / _____ ;

   half conscious

_____ / _____ ;

   half private (hospital room)

_____ / _____ .

1229

Build a word meaning:
presence of only half a heart (noun)

hemi/cardi/a

_____ / _____ / _____ ;

removal of half the stomach

_____ / _____ / _____ ;

hemi/gastr/ectomy
hemi/pleg/ia
(hemi/paralysis)
(You pronounce)

paralysis of half the body

_____ / _____ / ia .

1230

Build a word meaning:
half circular

semi/circular

_____ ;

half normal

semi/normal

_____ ;

half comatose

semi/comatose
(You pronounce)

_____ .

1231

Build a word with the literal meaning of:
half atrophy

hemi/a/troph/y

_____ / _____ / _____ / ;

half hypertrophy

hemi/hyper/troph/y

_____ / _____ / _____ / ;

half dystrophy

hemi/dys/troph/y
(You pronounce)

_____ / _____ / _____ / .

1232

con is a prefix that means **with.** Con/genit/al means born _____ .

with

1233

A child with con/genit/al cataracts is
*_____ cataracts.

born with

1234

There are many con/genit/al deformities. A child born with a lateral curvature of the spine has a
_____ / _____ / _____ scoliosis.

con/genit/al
congenital
kən jen′ i təl

answer column	
	1235
	Another way of saying born with deformity is to say congenital anomaly. A child born humpbacked has
congenital	a _____ anomaly.
	1236
	A child born with hydr/ophthalm/os has
congenital	_____ glaucoma.
	1237
	A child born with syphilis has
congenital	_____ syphilis.
	1238
	con —prefix—with
	sanguin/o —combining form—blood
	ity —noun suffix
	Using what you need of the above word parts, build a word meaning literally **with blood** or, in usage, **blood relationship.**
con/sanguin/ity consanguinity kon sang gwin′ i tē	_____ / _____ / _____
	1239
	Con/sanguin/ity is a relationship by descent from a common ancestor. The noun that expresses the relationship of cousins is
consanguinity	_____.
	1240
	The relationship of second cousins is that of
consanguinity	_____.
	1241
	sanguin/o means bloody. Build a word meaning pertaining to blood.
sanguin/al sang′ gwin əl	_____ / _____
	1242
	dis is a prefix that means **to free of, to separate,** or **to undo.** Dis/ease means literally
free of ease	** _____.

201

freed into

1243

To dis/sect is to cut a tissue or to undo it (into parts) for purposes of study. Analyze:

dis/sect

dissect

_____

dis/sect/ion

dissection

_____

dis/sect/ed
(You pronounce)

dissected

_____

1244

To dis/infect is to free of infective agents. Analyze:

dis/infect

disinfect _____

dis/infect/ant

disinfectant _____

dis/infect/ion

dis/infect/ed

disinfection _____

(You pronounce)

disinfected _____

1245

To dis/associate from reality is to be mentally ill. Analyze and check definitions:

dis/associate

disassociate _____

dis/sociate

dissociate _____

dis/sociated

dissociated _____

dis/sociation

dissociation _____

1246

to free of—to undo
with

dis is a prefix that means
_____ .
*

con is a prefix that means _____ .

Use the following chart to work Frames 1247 through 1253.

PREFIX	MEANING	
post	behind after	
ante	before forward	few usages
pre	before in front of	many usages

202

answer column	

after
behind

1247
Post/cibal means _____ meals.
Post/esophageal means _____ the esophagus.

before

in front of

1248
Pre/an/esthetic means _____ anesthesia.
Pre/hyoid means *_____ the hyoid bone.

before

forward

1249
Ante/pyretic means _____ the fever.
Ante/flexion means _____ bending.

post/nat/al
pre/nat/al
ante/nat/al
(You pronounce)

1250
Nat/al means birth. Think of the meaning while you analyze:

postnatal _____
prenatal _____
antenatal _____

post/febr/ile
post fē′ bril,
pōst feb′ rəl
ante/febr/ile
an tē fē′ brəl,
an tē feb′ rəl

1251
Febr/ile means pertaining to fever. Think of the meaning while you analyze:

postfebrile _____
antefebrile _____

post/operative
post/paralytic
post/uterine
post/partum
(You pronounce)

1252
Analyze:

postoperative _____
postparalytic _____
postuterine _____
postpartum _____

pre/operative
pre/paralytic
pre/frontal
pre/cancerous
(You pronounce)

1253
Analyze:

preoperative _____
preparalytic _____
prefrontal _____
precancerous _____

203

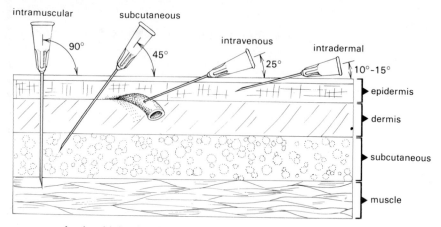

intramuscular

subcutaneous

90°

45°

intravenous

25°

intradermal

10°–15°

epidermis

dermis

subcutaneous

muscle

Angle of injection for parenteral administration of medication

answer column	
	1254
	Analyze:
ante/version	anteversion _____
ante/partum	antepartum _____
ante/position	anteposition _____
ante/location	antelocation _____
(You pronounce)	

1255

Mortem means death. What do these terms mean?
postmortem

after death

_____

antemortem

before death

_____

1256

into

within the abdomen

Intr/a means within. Intr/a-/abdominal means

* _____ .

1257

Intr/a/cellular means

within a cell

* _____ .

1258

Using intra and the adjectives ven/ous, spin/al, and
lumb/ar, build a word meaning:
within a vein

intravenous

_____ ;

within the spine

_____;

within the lumbar region

_____.

1259

Build an adjective meaning:
within an artery

_____;

within the cranium

_____;

within the bladder

_____.

1260

Build an adjective meaning:
within the skin _____;
within the duodenum

_____;

within the thoracic cavity

_____.

intra/derm/al

intra/duoden/al
intra/thorac/ic
(You pronounce)

Work Review Sheets 34 and 35.

1261

The following chart contains information about the formation of plurals from the singular. Use it to work Frames 1255 through 1279.

TO FORM PLURALS	
IF THE SINGULAR ENDING IS	THE PLURAL ENDING IS
a	ae (pronounce **ae** as ē)
us	i
um	a
ma	mata
on	a
is	es
ix	ices ⎫ The **word root is usually built**
ex	ices ⎬ from the plural form of words
ax	aces ⎭ ending in **ix, ex,** and **ax.** (e.g., radix, radic/es radic/otomy radic/i/form)

answer column

1262

Form the plural of:

	answer column
bursa	bursae *bûr' sē*
conjunctiva	conjunctivae *kon jungk tī' vē*
fossa	fossae *fos' ē*

bursa _____ *ae*

conjunctiva _____

fossa _____

1263

Give the singular of:

	answer column
vertebrae	vertebra *vûr' tə brə*
pleurae	pleura *ploor' ə*
corneae	cornea *kôr' nē ə*

vertebrae _____ *a*

pleurae _____

corneae _____

1264

Form the plural of:

	answer column
bacillus	bacilli *bə sil' ī*
bronchus	bronchi *brong' kī*
coccus	cocci *kok' sī*

bacillus _____ *i*

bronchus _____

coccus _____

1265

Give the singular of:

	answer column
foci	focus *fō' kəs*
loci	locus *lō' kəs*
nuclei	nucleus *noo' klē əs*

foci _____ *focus*

loci _____ *locus*

nuclei _____

1266

Form the plural of:

	answer column
atrium	atria *ā' trē ə*
delirium	deliria *di lir' ē ə*
ileum	ilea (You pronounce)

atrium _____

delirium _____

ileum _____

1267

Give the singular of:

	answer column
data	datum
bacteria	bacterium
ova	ovum (You pronounce)

data _____

bacteria _____

ova _____

206

carcinomata
kär sin ō′ mə tə
fibromata
fī brō′ mə tə
lipomata
li pō′ mə tə

1268

Form the plural of:

carninoma _____

fibroma _____

lipoma _____

*Note

---

enema
en′ ə mə
gumma
gum′ ə
stigma
stig′ mə

1269

Give the singular of:

enemata _____

gummata _____

stigmata _____

*Note

---

ganglia
gang′ glē ə
phenomena
fi nom′ ə nə
protozoa
prō tə zō′ ə

1270

Form the plural of:

ganglion _____

phenomenon _____

protozoon _____

---

zoon
zō′ on
encephalon
en sef′ ə lon
spermatozoon
spûr mə tō zō′ on

1271

Give the singular of:

zoa _____

encephala _____

spermatozoa _____

---

aponeuroses
ap ō noo rō′ sēz
diagnoses
dī əg nō′ sēz
pelves
pel′ vēz

1272

Form the plural of:

aponeurosis _____

diagnosis _____

pelvis _____

---

crisis
krī′ sis
naris
nair′ is
prognosis
prog nō′ sis

1273

Give the singular of:

crises _____

nares _____

prognoses _____

---

* This is formal plural usage. In practice you will see carcinomas, fibromas, lipomas, enemas, gums, stigmas as the plural forms.

1274

Form the plural of:

appendix _____ices_____

cortex _____

thorax _____

1275

Give the word root
that usually refers to:

the appendix _____

the cortex _____

the thorax _____

1276

The combining form of the word roots you just dis-
covered takes the **o**. They become:

appendix _____ / _____

cortic _____ / _____

thorac _____ / _____

1277

With this new knowledge that you found for yourself, build a word meaning:
inflammation of the appendix

appendic/itis
ə pen di sī′ tis

cortic/al
kôr′ ti kəl

thorac/o/centesis
thôr′ ə kō sen tē′ sis

_____ / _____;

pertaining to the cortex

_____ / _____;

surgical puncture of the thorax

_____ / ___ / _____.

1278

Form the plural of:

apex _____

fornix _____

varix _____

208

1279
Form the plural of:

sarcomata   sarcoma   _____

septa   septum   _____

radii   radius   _____

maxillae   maxilla   _____

(You pronounce)

Work Review Sheet 36.

---

free frame

1280
There are other ways for forming plurals. These apply to only a few words. When you meet these words and have a question about how their plural forms are built, consult a medical dictionary.

1281
The cervix is the neck of the uterus. The plural of

cervices   cervix is _____cervices_____ .

1282
Build the word root–combining form for cervix. The combining form takes **o**. The word root–combining

cervic/o   form is _____ / _____ .

1283
Build a word meaning:
     excision of the cervix

cervic/ectomy
sûr vi sek′ tə mē   _____ / _____ ;

     inflammation of the cervix

cervic/itis
sûr vi sīt′ is   _____ / _____ ;

     pertaining to the cervix

cervic/al
sûr′ vi kəl   _____ / _____ .

---

free frame

1284
cervic/o can mean the neck as well as the neck of the uterus. In usage you are not likely to confuse them. The next frame will make the point.

neck

neck

the neck of the uterus

1285

Cervic/o/facial means pertaining to the face and
_____. Cervic/o/brachial means pertaining to
the arm and _____.
Cervic/o/vesical means pertaining to the bladder
and

    *_____.

1286

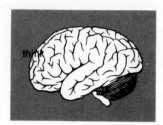

Use the following information to work Frames 1287
through 1314. If you have forgotten a word part,
remember, you may look back. The respiratory system is illustrated in the accompanying figure. Seeing
the parts as you work will make your work more
interesting.

Air enters the
    nose—nas/o (Remember rhin/o? Use nas/o in
                this work.)
goes to the
    pharynx—pharyng/o
to the
    larynx—laryng/o
to the
    trachea—trache/o
to the
    bronch/i—bronch/o
        (us)
to the
    part of the lung where it enters the bloodstream.
The lungs are covered by the
    pleura—pleur/o

The diaphragm (phren/o)- is a muscle that causes inhalation and exha-
lation.The phrenic nerve enervates the diaphragm.

1287

nose

Nas/o/antr/itis means inflammation of the antrum
and the _____.

1288

nose

Nas/o/ment/al means pertaining to the chin and

_____.

210

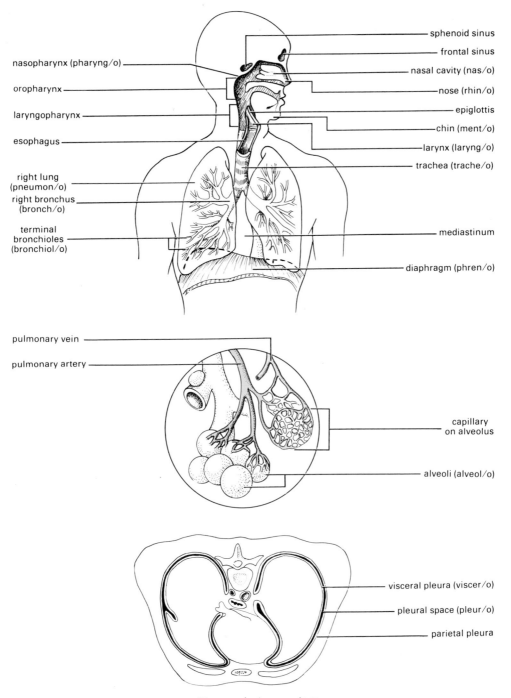

nasopharynx (pharyng/o)
oropharynx
laryngopharynx
esophagus
right lung (pneumon/o)
right bronchus (bronch/o)
terminal bronchioles (bronchiol/o)

sphenoid sinus
frontal sinus
nasal cavity (nas/o)
nose (rhin/o)
epiglottis
chin (ment/o)
larynx (laryng/o)
trachea (trache/o)
mediastinum
diaphragm (phren/o)

pulmonary vein
pulmonary artery

capillary on alveolus
alveoli (alveol/o)

visceral pleura (viscer/o)
pleural space (pleur/o)
parietal pleura

The respiratory system

1289
Build a word meaning:
pertaining to the nose _____/_____;
inflammation of the nose

_____/_____;

instrument to examine the nose

_____/_____/_____.

1290
Build a word (you may use your dictionary if necessary) meaning:
inflammation of nose and pharynx
_____/_____/_____;
pertaining to the nasal and frontal bones
_____/_____/_____;
pertaining to the nose and lacrimal duct
_____/_____/_____.

1291
Nas/o/pharyng/eal means pertaining to the
*_____.

1292
A pharyng/o/lith is a calculus in the wall of the
_____.

1293
A pharyng/o/myc/osis is a fungus disease of the
_____.

1294
Build a word meaning:
inflammation of the pharynx

_____/_____;

herniation of the pharynx
_____/_____/_____;
incision of the pharynx

_____/_____.

212

...

answer column	**1295** Build a word meaning (you put in diagonals): disease of the pharynx
	_____ ;
pharyng/o/path/y pharyng/o/plast/y pharyng/o/scop/e	surgical repair of the pharynx
	_____ ;
(You pronounce—review Frames 620 through 628)	instrument to examine the pharynx
	_____ .
	1296 **laryng/o** is used to build words that refer to the larynx. The larynx contains the vocal cords. When referring to the organ of sound, use
laryng/o	_____ / _____ .
laryng/itis laryngitis lar in jī′ tis	**1297** Form a word that means inflammation of the larynx. _____ / _____
laryng/algia laryngalgia lar in gal′ jē ə	**1298** After a bad cold, a patient may have laryng/itis with accompanying pain. Pain in the larynx is called _____ / _____ .
laryngostomy	**1299** Anything that obstructs the flow of air from the nose to the larynx may call for creating a new opening, or a _____ .
laryng/otomy laryngotomy lar ing got′ ə mē	**1300** When a **temporary opening** is wanted into the larynx, the surgical procedure is a laryng/**otomy**. An incision into the larynx is called a _____ / _____ .
laryngotomy (or laryngostomy)	**1301** When a patient has pneumonia and a freer flow of air is desired, the surgeon may incise the larynx and thus do a _____ .

Remember the "**g**" rule for pronunciation.

213

answer column

herniation of the larynx

1302
A laryng/o/cele is a
** _____ .

1303
Build a word meaning:
  any disease of the larynx

laryngopathy

  _____ ;

  instrument used to examine the larynx

laryngoscope

  _____ ;

laryngospasm
(You pronounce)

  spasm of the larynx

  _____ .

---

a condition of the trachea
  with pus formation
  (in your own words)

1304
Trache/o/py/osis means ** _____
_____ .

1305
Trache/orrhagia means ** _____

hemorrhage from the
  trachea

_____ .

1306
Build a word meaning:
  pain in the trachea

trachealgia
trā kē al′ jē ə

  _____ / _____ ;

tracheotomy
trā kē ot′ ə mē

  incision into the trachea

  _____ / _____ ;

tracheocele
trā′ kē ō sēl

  herniation of the trachea

  _____ / _____ / _____ .

1307
Build a word meaning:
  examination of the trachea

tracheoscopy

  _____ ;

  pertaining to the trachea

tracheal
tracheolaryngotomy
(You pronounce)

  _____ ;

  incision of trachea and larynx

  _____ .

214

answer column

inflammation of the bronchi	**1308**
an instrument to examine the bronchi	Bronchitis means * _____. A bronchoscope is * _____.

1309

Build a word meaning:

calculus in a bronchus

bronch/o/lith
brong′ kō lith

_____ / ___ / _____ ;

bronch/o/scop/y
brong kos′ kə pē

examination of a bronchus (with instrument)

_____ / ___ / _____ / ___ ;

bronch/orrhagia
brong kō rā′ jē ə

bronchial hemorrhage

_____ / _____ .

1310

Build a word meaning:

bronchostomy

formation of a new opening into a bronchus

_____ ;

bronchospasm

spasm of a bronchus

_____ ;

bronchorrhaphy
(You pronounce)

suturing of a bronchus

_____ .

1311

Pleur/al means
 * _____.

pertaining to the pleura

Pleur/itis means
 * _____.

inflammation of the pleura

1312

Build a word meaning:

pain in the pleura

pleur/algia
ploo ral′ jē ə
pleur/o/dynia
ploor ō din′ ē ə

_____ / _____ or

_____ / ___ / _____ ;

pleur/o/centesis
ploor ō sen tē′ sis

surgical puncturing of the pleura

_____ / ___ / _____ .

215

answer column

1313
Build a word meaning:
pertaining to the pleura and viscer/a
______________________;
calculus in the pleura
______________________;
excision of part of the pleura
______________________.

pleurovisceral
pleurolith
pleurectomy
(You pronounce)

1314
Look up the word pleurisy. Read all your dictionary has to say about this disease.

1315
The phrenic nerve controls the diaphragm. The word root–combining form for diaphragm is **phren/o.** Pleg/ia is the word root–combining form for paralysis. Paralysis of the diaphragm is
______________ / / ______________.

phren/o/pleg/ia
phrenoplegia
fren ō plē′ jē ə

1316
Removal of a portion of the phrenic nerve is a ______________________.

phren/ectomy
phrenectomy
fren ek′ tōm ē

1317
The word sinister means wicked or evil. The Latin word sinister means **left** or **left-handed.** In medieval times when superstition was rampant, the majority of the people (who were right-handed) considered left-handed people cursed by the devil. Hence these unfortunate few people became the personification of evil. This is how sinister found its common, contemporary meaning.

a little story frame

1318
In medicine you go back to the original meaning of sinister to find the word root–combining form, sinistr/o, which means ______________.

left

1319
Sinistr/ad means toward the ______________.

left

answer column	
	1320
	Using sinistr/o build a word meaning:
	pertaining to the left
sinistr/al	
sin′ is trəl	_____ / _____ ;
sinistr/o/cardi/a	displacement of the heart to the left
sin is trō kär′ dē ə	_____ / ___ / _____ / ___ ;
sinistr/o/cerebr/al	pertaining to the left half of the cerebrum
sin is trō ser′ ə brəl	_____ / ___ / _____ / _____ .
	1321
	With manual and pedal, build a word meaning:
sinistromanual	left-handed _____ ;
sinistropedal	left-footed _____ .
(You pronounce)	
	1322
	The opposite of sinistr/o is dextr/o. Dextr/o means
right	_____ .
	~~1323~~
right	Dextr/ad means toward the ___*right*___ .
	1324
	Build a word meaning:
	pertaining to the right
dextr/al	
dek′ strəl	_____ / _____ ;
	displacement of the heart to the right
dextr/o/cardi/a	_____ / ___ / _____ / ___ ;
dek strō kär′ dē ə	
dextr/o/gastr/ia	displacement of the stomach to the right
dek strō gas′ trē ə	_____ / ___ / _____ / _____ .
	1325
	Refer to Frame 1321 if necessary, and build a word meaning:
	right-handed
dextromanual	_____ ;
dextropedal	right-footed
(You pronounce)	_____ .

217

answer column	
foot pod/o	**1326** Look up **podalgia.** Podalgia means pain in the _____. The new word root–combining form is _____ / ____ .
pod/iatrist podiatrist pō dī ə trist	**1327** Suffixes **iatrist** (noun) and **iatric** (adjective) are used to indicate medical professionals. A health professional responsible for care of conditions of the feet is a _____ / _____ .
spasm of the hand chir/o	**1328** Look up **chirospasm;** it means * _____ . The word root–combining form for hand is _____ / ____ .
pod/i/atric podiatric pōd ē a′ trik	**1329** A podiatrist provides _____ treatment.
chiro/plasty chiroplasty kī′ rō plas tē	**1330** Surgical repair of the hand is called _____ / _____
hands	**1331** Chiropractors use their hands to manipulate the body for therapy. In the adjective chiro/practic, the word root **chiro** means _____ .
iatrist	**1332** A psychiatrist is a medical doctor who specializes in diagnosing and treating mental disorders. _____ is the suffix used to indicate a medical professional.
psych/i/atric psychiatric si kē a′ trik	**1333** A psychiatrist provides _____ treatment.

answer column	

1334

Vas is a word meaning vessel. Vas/o is another word root–combining form for vessel. Vas/o/dilatation means enlarging the diameter of a

_____.

vessel

1335

Vas/o/constriction is the opposite of vas/o/dilatation.
Vas/o/constriction means ** _____

_____.

decreasing the size of
the diameter of a vessel

1336

Vas/o/motor is an adjective that refers to nerves that control the tone of the blood

_____ walls.

vessel

1337

Using vas/o build a word meaning:

pertaining to a vessel _____/_____;
spasm of a vessel

_____/___/_____;

crushing of a vessel

_____/___/_____.

(with forceps for hemorrhage)

vas/al
vā′ səl, vā′ zəl
vas/o/spasm
vas′ ō spaz əm,
vā′ zō spaz əm
vas/o/tripsy
vas′ ō trip sē,
vā′ zō trip sē

1338

Look at the words used in your dictionary beginning with vas or vas/o. Only six of them use the common medical forms and could be confused with angi/o. The three words in Frame 1339 refer to the vas deferens only—no other vessel. The vas deferens is shown in the illustration on page 92.

Examine the words in
your dictionary to see
which ones begin with
vas/o

1339

Build a word meaning:
incision into the vas deferens

_____/_____;

suture of the vas deferens

_____/_____;

vas/otomy
vas ot′ ə mē

vas/orrhaphy
vas ôr′ ə fē

219

vas/ostomy vas os′ tə mē	making a new opening into the vas deferens _____/_____;
vas/ectomy vas ek′ tə mē	removal of a segment of the vas deferens _____/_____.

1340

The word root-combining form that refers to tissue is **hist/o**. Hist/o/lys/is is the destruction of

tissue

_____.

1341

tissue

A substance that is hist/o/genous is a substance that is made by a _____.

1342

hist/o/log/y
his tol′ ə je

hist/o/log/ist
his tol′ ə jist

hist/oma
(You pronounce)

Build a word meaning:
   the study of tissue

_____/_____/_____/_____;

   one who studies tissues

_____/_____/_____/_____;

   a tumor composed of tissue

_____/_____.

1343

hist/o/blast
hist/o/cyt/e
hist/oid
(You pronounce)

Build a word meaning:
   an embryonic tissue (cell)

_____/_____/_____;

   a tissue cell   _____/_____/_____/_____;

   resembling tissue   _____/_____.

1344

new

ne/o in words means new. Ne/o/genesis means re-generation of _____ tissue.

1345

new
new

Ne/o/nat/al refers to the _____ born. A ne/o/plasm is a tumor or _____ growth (formation—plasm/o).

220

1346

Ne/o/plasm refers to any kind of tumor or new growth. A nonmalignant tumor is called a

| ne/o/plasm |
| neoplasm |
| nē′ ō plaz əm |

benign _____ / _____ / _____.

1347

A neoplasm may also be a malignant tumor. Carcinoma is a _____. A melanoma is also a _____.

| neoplasm |
| neoplasm |

1348

A sarcoma is also a _____.

| neoplasm |

1349

Build a word meaning:

ne/o/cyt/e	new cell _____ / _____ / _____ / e ;
ne/o/path/y	any new disease _____ / _____ / _____ / y ;
ne/o/phob/ia	abnormal fear of new things
(You pronounce)	_____ / _____ / _____.

Work Review Sheets 37 and 38.

1350

There are two combining forms that mean night. One is **noct/i.** Noct/i/luca are microscopic marine animals that make the ocean glow during the

| night |

_____.

1351

Those of you who have studied music know that a noct/urne is dreamy music, sometimes called

| night |

_____ music.

1352

Noct/ambulism literally means walking at night. Sleepwalking is what you mean when you use the

| noct/ambul/ism |
| nok tam′ byoo liz əm |

word _____ / _____.

1353

Noctambulism can occur at any age, but childhood is the most common age for

| noctambulism |

_____.

221

1354

People are not really asleep when they sleepwalk. They appear to be asleep but are really suppressing the memory of what they do. They are indulging in

noctambulism

_____ .

1355

The other combining form for night is **nyct/o.** Nyct/algia means pain during the _____ .

night

1356

Nyct/albumin/ur/ia means the presence of albumin in the urine only during the _____ .

night

1357

Nyct/al/opia means night blindness or difficulty in seeing at night. Vitamin A is associated with night vision. Lack of vitamin A in the diet is one cause of _____ .

nyctalopia
nik tə lō′ pē ə

1358

Nyct/al/opia has several causes. Retinal fatigue from exposure to very bright light is a cause of

nyctalopia

_____ .

1359

Retinitis pigmentosa is another cause of

nyctalopia

_____ .

1360

Using noct/i and nyct/o build two words that mean:
abnormal fear of night

nyct/o/phob/ia

_____ / / _____ / _____

noct/i/phob/ia

_____ / / _____ / _____ ;

unusual attraction to the night

nyct/o/phil/ia
noct/i/phil/ia
(You pronounce)

_____ / / _____ / _____

_____ / / _____ / _____ .

1361

Noct/uria means excessive urination during the night. Another word that means the same thing is

nyct/ur/ia
nik tyoor′ ē ə

_____ / _____ .

222

1362

Two words that mean excessive urination during the night are:

nyct/uria

_____ / _____

noct/uria

_____ / _____

1363

ankyl/o means stiff or not movable. Ankylosed means stiffened. Ankyl/o/blephar/on means adhesions resulting in

immovable eyelids

** _____ .

1364

Ankyl/osis is a condition of

stiffness

_____ .

Use the following chart to build words through Frame 1373.

COMBINING FORM	WITH NOUN ENDING
aden/o	aden/ia
cardi/o	cardi/a
cheil/o	cheil/ia
dactyl/o	dactyl/ia
dent/o	dent/ia
derm/o	derm/a
	/ia
gastr/o	gastr/ia
gloss/o	gloss/ia
onych/o	onych/ia
ophthalm/o	ophthalm/ia
ot/o	ot/ia
phag/o	phag/ia
pneumon/o	pneumon/ia
proct/o	proct/ia
urethr/o	urethr/a

1365

Ankyl/o/stom/a means lockjaw (stiff jaw). Build a word meaning (**remember, you may look back**): adhesions of lips (immovable lips)

ankyl/o/cheil/ia

_____ / _____ / _____ ;

223

ankyl/o/proct/ia

ankyl/o/phob/ia
(You pronounce)

closure (immobility) of the anus

_____ / / _____ / ___ ;

abnormal fear of ankylosis

_____ / / _____ / ___ .

1366
Build a word meaning:
tongue tied (stiff tongue)

ankyl/o/gloss/ia

_____ / / _____ / ___ ;

adhesions of fingers (immovable fingers)

ankyl/o/dactyl/ia

_____ / / _____ / ___ .

1367

noun

ia is a _____ (noun/adjective/verb) ending.

1368
Do you remember the origin of o/o/phor/o (Frame 602)? O/o/phor/o refers to the organ that

bears

_____ ova.

1369
Ex/o/phor/ia refers to imbalance of the muscle

carries or bears

that _____ the eye outward (wall eye). Es/o/phor/ia refers to imbalance of the mus-

carries or bears

cle that _____ the eye mesially (cross eye).

1370
The instrument that measures the tone and pull of the eye-carrying (bearing) muscles is a

phor/o/meter
phorometer
fôr om′ ə tər

_____ / / _____ .

1371
Hyper/phor/ia results when an eye muscle carries

hypo/phor/ia
hypophoria
hī pō fôr′ ē ə

one eye upward. When one eye turns downward, we call it _____ / / _____ .

1372
Dys/phor/ia means a feeling of depression—you carry with you an ill (bad) feeling. The word that

eu/phor/ia
yōō fôr′ ē ə

means feeling of well-being is

_____ / / _____ .

224

1373

When your diet is good, you have enough rest, and the world is a wonderful place to be, you are enjoying the state of _____.

euphoria

1374

The study of people, insects, or animals that carry (bear) disease is called

_____ / _____ / _____ / _____.

phor/o/log/y
fôr ol′ ə jē

1375

Stasis is a word meaning **stopping** or **controlling.** To say that you control an organ or what that organ produces, use the combining form for the organ (or product), plus the word

_____.

stasis
(You pronounce)

1376

Fungistasis is a condition in which the growth of fungi is _____.

stopped or controlled

1377

Chol/e/stasis means

**_____.

(Refer to Frame 512 if necessary.)

control or stopping of
bile secretion

1378

Read Frame 1375 again. Build a word meaning:
  controlling the small intestine

_____ / _____ / _____;

  stopping the formation of pus

_____ / _____ / _____.

enter/o/stasis
enterostasis
en tə ros′ tə sis
py/o/stasis
pyostasis
pī os′ tə sis

1379

Build a word meaning:
  controlling the flow of blood

_____ / _____ / _____;

  checking flow in the veins

_____ / _____ / _____;

  checking flow in the arteries

_____ / _____ / _____.

hemostasis
hē mos′ tə sis
phlebostasis or veno-
  stasis
fli bos′ tə sis
arteriostasis
är tir′ ē os′ tə sis

225

1380

Schiz/o, schist/o, and schis/o are all combining forms that have a complicated evolution from Greek. They mean split (cleft or fissure). Analyze the following words and check meanings:

schiz/o/phren/ia
skit zō frē' nē ə
schiz/o/phas/ia
schiz/o/cyt/e

schizophrenia _____

schizophasia _____

schizocyte _____

1381

schist/o/gloss/ia
skis to glos' ē ə,
shis tō glos' ē ə
schist/o/cyt/e
schist/o/thorax

Analyze the following words and check meanings:

schistoglossia _____

schistocyte _____

schistothorax _____

1382

palat/o/schis/is
pal ə tos' ki sis
uran/o/schis/is
yoor ə nos' ki sis
rach/i/schis/is
rə kis' ki sis

Analyze the following words and check meanings:

palatoschisis _____

uranoschisis _____

rachischisis _____

1383

In your dictionary, read about the disease schisto-somiasis and Schistosoma. Schistosomiasis is a very important disease in terms of world health. Because of increased worldwide travel all people should be concerned with the disease,

schist/o/som/iasis

_____ / / _____ / _____.

1384

Learn the words involving the combining forms for "split" that you need to know. Surely schizophrenia will be one of them. Use your dictionary to under-stand the words you (or your teacher) decide you should learn. Schiz/o, schist/o, and schis/o mean

split

_____.

Use the labels on the following drawing plus your dictionary to work Frames 1385 through 1422.

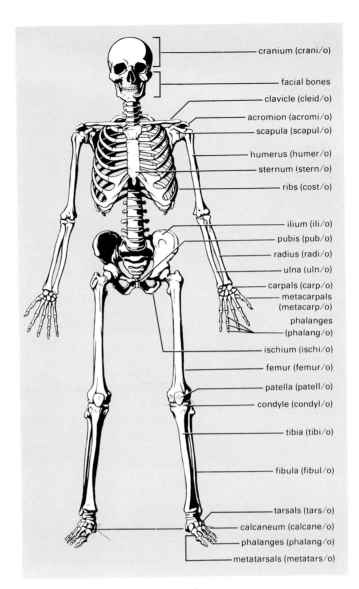

cranium (crani/o)

facial bones

clavicle (cleid/o)

acromion (acromi/o)

scapula (scapul/o)

humerus (humer/o)

sternum (stern/o)

ribs (cost/o)

ilium (ili/o)

pubis (pub/o)

radius (radi/o)

ulna (uln/o)

carpals (carp/o)

metacarpals (metacarp/o)

phalanges (phalang/o)

ischium (ischi/o)

femur (femur/o)

patella (patell/o)

condyle (condyl/o)

tibia (tibi/o)

fibula (fibul/o)

tarsals (tars/o)

calcaneum (calcane/o)

phalanges (phalang/o)

metatarsals (metatars/o)

The skeletal system

calcanea
kal kā′ nē ə

1385
Locate the calcaneum. The plural of calcaneum is

_____ .

calcane

1386
From calcaneum and calcanea, derive the word root for the heel. _____

227

1387

In your medical dictionary, look at the words beginning with calcane. Derive the combining form that is used in words that refer to the heel.

calcane/o

_____ /

1388

Close your dictionary. Now build a word meaning:

    pertaining to the heel

calcane/al
calcaneal
kal kā′ nē əl
calcane/o/dynia
calcaneodynia
kal kā′ nē ō din′ ē ə

    _____ / _____ ;

    pain in the heel

    _____ / ___ / _____ .

1389

heel

Calcane/o in a word refers to the _____ .

1390

carpi

Locate the carpus. The plural of carpus is _____ .

1391

carp

From carpus and carpi, derive a word root that refers to the wrist. It is _____ .

1392

Look at the words (in your medical dictionary) that begin with carp. The combining form that is used in words about the wrist is _____ / ___ .

carp/o

1393

Close your dictionary. Build a word meaning:

    pertaining to the wrist (adjective)

carpal
kär′ pəl

carpoptosis
kär pop tō′ sis

carpectomy
kär pek′ tə mē

    _____ / ___ ;

    prolapse of the wrist

    _____ / ___ / _____ ;

    excision of all or part of the wrist

    _____ / _____ .

1394

wrist

Carp/o in a word refers to the _____ .

228

1395

You are now finding your own word root–combining forms. Feels good, doesn't it? Let's do some more.

---

congratulations!

1396

Locate the ischium. The plural of ischium is

_____.

ischia

1397

From ischium and ischia, derive a word root that refers to the part of the hip bone on which the body rests when sitting. The word root is

_____.

ischi (Tail bone)

1398

Look up words that begin with ischi. The combining form that is used in words to refer to the ischium is

_____ / _____.

ischi/o

1399

In your dictionary, find a word meaning:
  pertaining to the ischium and rectum
  ischi/o / rect /al ;

  neuralgic pain in the hip (synonym is sciatica)
  ischi/o / neuralg / ia ;

  pertaining to the ischium and pubis
  ischi/o / pub /ic .

ischi/o/rect/al
is kē ō rek′ təl

ischi/o/neuralg/ia
is′ kē ō noo ral′ jē ə

ischi/o/pub/ic
is kē ō pyoo′ bik

1400

Close your dictionary. Build a word meaning:
  pertaining to the ischium

  _____ / _____;

  herniation through the ischium

  _____ / ___ / _____.

ischi/al
is′ kē əl

ischi/o/cele
is′ kē ō sēl

1401

(ischi/o) in a word refers to the part of the hip bone known as the _____.

ischium
is′ kē əm

229

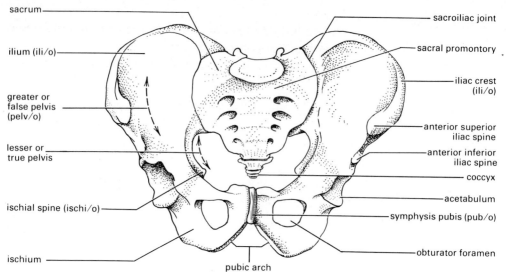

sacrum

ilium (ili/o)

greater or
false pelvis
(pelv/o)

lesser or
true pelvis

ischial spine (ischi/o)

ischium

sacroiliac joint

sacral promontory

iliac crest
(ili/o)

anterior superior
iliac spine

anterior inferior
iliac spine

coccyx

acetabulum

symphysis pubis (pub/o)

obturator foramen

pubic arch

The pelvis—anterior view

answer column	
pubes pyōō′ bēz	**1402** Locate the pubis. The plural of pubis is _____.
pub/o (used most often) or pubi/o	**1403** The word root–combining form used in words about the pubis is _____/____. (Don't forget your dictionary.)

pub/ic
pyōō′ bik
 	
pub/o/femor/al
pyōō bō fem′ ər əl
	1404
	Close your dictionary. Using pub/o, build a word meaning:
	  pertaining to the pubis _____/_____;
	  pertaining to the pubis and femur
	  _____/___/_____/_____.

pubis	**1405** **pub/o** in a word refers to the _____.
stern/o	**1406** Locate the sternum. The word root–combining form for sternum is _____/___.

1407

You did that one all alone! With your dictionary still open, find a word meaning:

pertaining to the sternum and pericardium

__sternopericardial__ ;

pertaining to the sternum and ribs

__sternocostal__ .

1408

Close the dictionary. Build a word meaning:

pertaining to the sternum

__sternial__ ;

pain in the sternum

__stern/algia__ or

__ / /__ .

1409

__stern/o__ in a word makes you think of the
_____, which is the __breastbone__ .

1410

Locate the phalanges. They are the **_____
_____ .

bones of the fingers
and toes (can omit
fingers or toes)

1411

The word root for phalanges is
_____ .

1412

Build a word meaning:

inflammation of phalanges

_____ / _____ ;

excision of a phalanx (singular)

_____ / _____ .

1413

Locate the acromion. It is a projection of the
__scapul__ _____ (dictionary if necessary).

231

1414

The word root–combining form for the acromion is

acromi/o

_____ / _____ .

1415

Find a word in your dictionary meaning:
  pertaining to the acromion

acromi/al
ə krō′ mē əl
acromi/o/humer/al
acromiohumeral
ə krō′ mē ō hyoo′ mər əl

_____ / _____ ;

pertaining to the acromion and humerus

_____ / _____ / _____ / _____ .

1416

Look at Frame 1415. Can it start you looking for another word root–combining form? Try. It is

humer/o

_____ / _____ .

1417

humer/o is used in words to refer to the bone of the upper arm, which is named the

humerus

_____ .

1418

Find three words in your dictionary that begin with humer or humer/o. They are:

(pick three out of four)

humeral
humeroradial
humeroscapular
humeroulnar

_____

_____

_____

1419

Could Frame 1418 start you building other word root–combining forms? Well, it isn't necessary, but you may if you like.

It could get to be a
  never-ending thing,
  couldn't it?

1420

Refer back to the drawing of the skeleton. Locate a condyle. A condyle is a rounded process that occurs on many bones. The word root for condyle is _____ .

condyl

1421

Build a word meaning:

excision of a condyle

_____ / _____ ;

resembling a condyle

_____ / _____ ;

above a condyle

_____ epi ____ / _____ .

1422

Condyl/ar is an adjective meaning pertaining to a

_____ .

1423

The plural of ganglion is ganglia. A ganglion is a collection of nerve cell bodies. Now that you have a system, form the word root–combining form for ganglion. _____ / ____

1424

Practice using the singular and plural of gangli/o words correctly by working Frames 1424 through 1428. The singular noun built from gangli/o is

_____ .

1425

The plural form of the noun built from gangli/o is

_____ .

1426

There is a mass of gray matter beneath the third ventricle called the basal optic _____ .

1427

The main cerebral nerve centers are called the cerebral _____ .

1428

Any one of three neural masses found in the cervical region is called a cervical _____ , whereas all three are referred to as the cervical _____ .

Work Review Sheets 39 and 40.

233

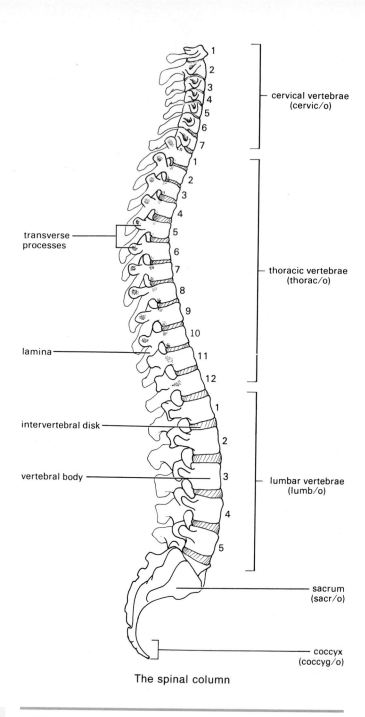

The spinal column

answer column

1429

You are now ready to find word roots and their combining forms by another method. Look up the word spine in your dictionary. A synonym for spine is

_____.

backbone

spine

1430

Look in your dictionary for words beginning with rach. Rach is the word root for

_____ .

---

rach/itis
rə kī′ tis or
spondyl/itis
spon di lī′ tis

1431

There are two word roots that mean spine. One is rach, the other is spondyl. Build a word that means inflammation of the spine

_____ / _____ .

---

spine

1432

Words beginning with rachi/o or spondyl/o refer to the

_____ .

---

rachi/algia
rā kē al′ jē ə

rachi/otomy
rā kē ot′ ə mē

1433

Using rachi/o, build a word meaning:
   spine pain

_____ / _____ ;

   incision into the spine

_____ / _____ .

---

rachi/o/dynia
rā kē ō din′ ē ə

rachi/o/meter
rā kē om′ ə tər

rachi/o/pleg/ia
rā kē ō plē′ jē ə

1434

Using rachi/o, build a word meaning:
   a synonym for rachialgia

_____ / _____ / _____ ;

   instrument to measure spinal curvature

_____ / _____ / _____ ;

   spinal paralysis

_____ / _____ / _____ / _____ .

---

rach/i/schis/is
rə kis′ kis is

rach/itis
(You pronounce)

1435

In the same manner using rach/i, build a word meaning:
   fissure of the spine (split spine)

_____ / _____ / _____ / _____ is ;

   inflammation of the spine

_____ / _____ .

235

spine	**1436** Words beginning with rach/i or rachi/o refer to the _____. See "Case Study: Radiology Report" on opposite page.
	1437 **ophthalm/o** is used in words to mean eye. Ophthalm/itis means
inflammation of the eye	* _____.
pertaining to the eye	Ophthalm/ic means * _____.
pain in the eye	**1438** Ophthalm/algia and ophthalm/o/dyn/ia both mean * _____.
practice pronouncing look at the ph th	**1439** Before building words with this root, be sure you have the **phth** order of o**phth**alm/o straight. Pronounce it **off thalm o.**
ophthalm/o/cele ophthalmocele of thal′ mō sēl ophthalm/o/meter ophthalmometer of thal mom′ ə ter	**1440** Build a word meaning: herniation of an eye (abnormal protrusion) _____ / _____ / _____ ; instrument for measuring the eye _____ / _____ / _____ .
ophthalm/o/path/y	**1441** Build a word meaning: any eye disease _____ / __ / _____ / __ ; plastic surgery of eye
ophthalm/o/plast/y	_____ / __ / _____ / __ ;
ophthalm/o/pleg/ia (You pronounce)	paralysis of the eye _____ / __ / _____ / __ .
ophthalm/o/log/ist	**1442** Ophthalmology is the medical specialty dealing with eye disease. We call the physician who practices this specialty an _____ / __ / _____ / __ .

236

CASE STUDY: RADIOLOGY REPORT

REASON FOR EXAM: Lumbar myelogram.

ADDITIONAL HISTORY: Left-side pain with left foot drop.

INTERPRETATION: *Lumbosacral Spine:* AP, lateral, and oblique views obtained of the lumbosacral spine show minimal dextroscoliosis of the upper lumbar spine. There are changes of degenerative disk disease between L1–L2 and L3–L4. Also, a small amount of residual contrast is noted in the lower thecal sac. *Lumbar Myelogram:* Contrast (Isovue-M200) was injected into the lumbar subarachnoid space between L3 and L4. Multiple films were obtained during fluoroscopy, followed by overhead filming. The thecal sac is fairly well opacified. The nerve roots are symmetrically filled. No evidence of edema or obliteration of the nerve root sleeve is noted. There is a vague impression on the thecal sac from the right lateral and anterior aspect at L4–L5. The cauda equina region appears normal.

IMPRESSION: 1. No definite evidence of disk herniation.
2. Vague impression on the thecal sac from the right lateral anterior aspect suggests the possibility of facet hypertrophy. The other possibility is bulging disk. However, the patient's symptoms are on the left side. In view of the findings, CT (computed tomography) scan at this level is suggested.

---

answer column	
	1443
	Ophthalm/o/scop/y is the examination of the interior of the eye. The instrument used for this examination is an
ophthalm/o/scop/e	_____ / / _____ / ___ .

	1444
	opia is a suffix denoting vision. Cyan/opia is a defect in vision that causes objects to appear blue. Form a word meaning:
xanth/opia	
zan thō′ pē ə	yellow vision _____ / _____
chlor/opia	
klor ō′ pē ə	green vision _____ / _____
erythr/opia	
er i thrō′ pē ə	red vision _____ / _____

	1445
	Look up the following terms and note the type of vision they are describing.
near-sightedness	myopia * _____
far-sightedness	hyperopia * _____
loss of accommodation	presbyopia * _____
double vision	diplopia * _____

237

1446

Blephar/o/ptosis means prolapse of an eyelid. The word root–combining form for eyelid is

blephar/o

_____ / _____ .

1447

Blepharedema means swelling of the

eyelid

_____ .

eyelid

blephar/o seen anywhere makes you think of the

_____ .

1448

Blephar/edema means swelling of the eyelid. Build a word that means:

    inflammation of an eyelid

blephar/itis
blef ə rī′ tis

_____ / _____ ;

blephar/otomy
blef ə rot′ ə mē

    incision of an eyelid

_____ / _____ .

1449

Build a word that means:

    surgical repair of eyelid

blephar/o/plast/y
blef′ ə rō plas tē

_____ / _____ / _____ / _____ ;

blephar/o/spasm
blef′ ə rō spaz əm

    twitching of an eyelid

_____ / _____ / _____ ;

blephar/o/ptosis
blef ər op tō′ sis

    prolapse of an eyelid

_____ / _____ / _____ .

1450

Look up cornea in your dictionary. Look at the words in our dictionary that begin with **corne.** A word root–combining form for cornea is

corne/o

_____ / _____ .

1451

While thinking of the meaning, analyze:

corne/itis
kôr nē ī′ tis

    corneitis _____ / _____

corne/o/ir/itis
kôr nē ō ī rī′ tis

    corneoiritis

_____ / _____ / _____ / _____

corne/o/scler/a
kôr nē ō sklir′ ə

    corneosclera

_____ / _____ / _____ / _____

238

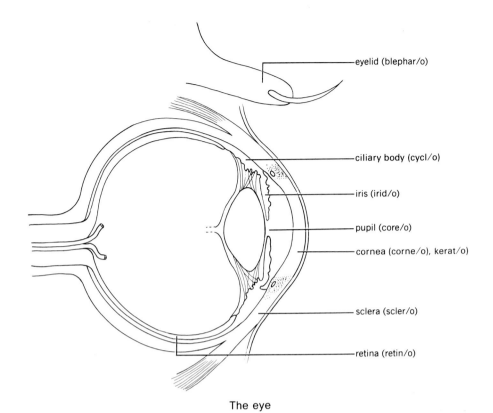

eyelid (blephar/o)

ciliary body (cycl/o)

iris (irid/o)

pupil (core/o)

cornea (corne/o), kerat/o)

sclera (scler/o)

retina (retin/o)

The eye

answer column

ir
scler

1452
From the preceding frame find two other word roots that match labels on your drawing. They are _____ and _____.

sclera
sklir′ ə

1453
Look up the first word in your dictionary beginning with scler. It is _____.

1454
Read what the sclera is. Does the word root plus the meaning of the Greek word from which it is derived suggest an already familiar combining form

scler/o
hard

to you? It is _____ / _____, which means _____.

1455
The sclera of the eye is the "hard" outer coat of the eye. Build a word meaning:
    pertaining to the sclera (adjective)

scler/al
sklir′ əl

_____ / _____;

239

scler/ectomy
skli rek′ tə mē

scler/ostomy
skli ros′ tə mē

iris
ī′ ris

ir/itis

corne/o/ir/itis

scler/o/ir/itis
(You pronounce)

irides
ir′ i dēz, ī′ ri dēz

irid/o

irid/o/cele
i rid′ ō sēl, ī rid′ ō sel

---

excision of the sclera (or part)

_____ / _____;

formation of an opening into the sclera

_____ / _____.

1456

Go back to the other word root you found in Frame 1452. With it in mind, find the part of the eye (on your drawing) to which it refers. This is the

_____.

1457

Look up "iris" in your dictionary. **ir** is one word root for the iris. It is very limited in use. It is always used to express inflammation, so you can see it is important if limited in use.

1458

With the information in Frame 1457 and the word root you found, build a word meaning:
    inflammation of the iris

_____ / _____;

    inflammation of the cornea and iris

_____ / _____ / _____;

    inflammation of the sclera and iris

_____ / _____ / _____.

1459

In your dictionary find the plural of **iris.** It is

_____.

1460

With your dictionary, find the combining form for irid. It is _____ / _____.

1461

Using irid/o build a word meaning:
    herniation of the iris

_____ / _____ / _____;

240

irid/algia
ir i dal′ jē ə, ī ri dal′ jē ə
irid/ectomy
ir i dek′ tə mē,
ī ri dek′ tə mē

pain in the iris

_____/_____;

excision of part of the iris

_____/_____.

1462
Build a word meaning (you insert the diagonals):
   prolapse of the iris

irid/o/ptosis

_____;

   softening of the iris

irid/o/malac/ia

_____;

irid/orrhexis
(You pronounce)

   rupture of the iris

_____.

1463
There are two words to express paralysis of the iris.

iridoplegia

They are _____/___/_____/_____
and

iridoparalysis
(You pronounce)

_____/___/_____.

1464
The following forms make you think of:

iris

   ir   _____

iris

   irid/o _____

sclera (hard)

   scler/o _____

cornea

   corne/o _____

1465
Look up **retina** in your dictionary. Read about the retina. Look at the words beginning with retin in your dictionary. The word root—combining form for words about the retina is

retin/o

_____/___.

1466
Build a word meaning:
   pertaining to the retina

retinal
ret′ i nəl

_____/___;

241

inflammation of the retina

_____/_____ ;

fixation of a detached retina

_____/_____ .

1467

The instrument used to examine the retina is the

_____/___/_____/___ . The

process of examining the retina is

_____/___/_____/___ .

1468

The pupil in the eye is the opening in the iris through which light passes. Identify the pupil in the illustration of the eye on page 239. The word root for pupil is **cor.**

1469

The combining form for pupil is cor/e. Build a word meaning:

    pupil misplaced

_____/_____ ;

destruction of the pupil

corectas/ia
     /is
kôr ek tā′ zhə

_____/___/_____/___ ;

dilatation (stretching) of the pupil

_____/_____/___ .

1470

cor/e/o is also used as a combining form for **pupil.** Using core/o, build a word meaning:

    instrument for measuring the pupil

_____ ;

measurement of the pupil

_____ ;

plastic surgery of the pupil

_____ .

1471

Whether cor/e or cor/e/o is used, the word root for pupil of the eye is _____ .

242

1472

You have already learned one word root for cornea.
It is _____. Another word root for cornea is
kerat and it is the more commonly used form.

corne

1473

The word root most commonly used for cornea
is _____. The combining form is

kerat

kerat/o

_____/_____ .

1474

Using kerat/o build a word meaning:
    dilatation of the cornea

kerat/ectas/ia(is)
ker ə tek tā′ zhə

_____/_____ ;

    herniation through the cornea

kerat/o/cele
ker′ ə tō sēl

_____/_____/_____ ;

    plastic operation of the cornea (corneal trans-
    plant)

kerat/o/plast/y
ker′ ə tō plas tē

_____/_____/_____/_____ .

1475

Build a word meaning:
    incision of the cornea

kerat/otomy

_____/_____ ;

    corneal rupture

kerat/orrhexis

_____/_____ ;

    inflammation of cornea and sclera

kerat/o/scler/itis
(You pronounce)

_____/_____/_____/_____ .

1476

The word root-combining form for **ciliary body** is
cycl/o. Look up the ciliary body in your dictionary
or an anatomy book and understand what it is.

think

1477

Turn to cycl/o words in your dictionary. Find a word
meaning:
    paralysis of the ciliary body (noun)

cycl/o/pleg/ia
sī klō plē′ jē ə

_____/_____/_____/_____ ;

243

cycl/o/pleg/ic
sī klō plē′ jik

paralysis of the ciliary body (adjective)

_____ / ___ / _____ / _____.

1478

Good work—now, remember them

Cycloplegia and cycloplegic are words used often in the practice of ophthalmology. For that reason write them both several times.

_____   _____

_____   _____

_____   _____

_____   _____

1479

The following forms make you think of:

retina

     retin/o _____

pupil

     cor/e _____

pupil

     cor/e/o _____

cornea

     kerat/o _____

ciliary body

     cycl/o _____

1480

Look at the drawing of the lacrimal apparatus. The word root that you see immediately is

lacrim

                                           _____.

1481

tears

Look up lacrim/al in your dictionary. Lacrimal is a word that means pertaining to _____.

1482

lacrimal
lak′ ri məl

The gland that secretes tears is the

_____ gland.

1483

lacrimal

The sac that collects lacrimal fluid is the

_____ sac.

1484

nas/o/lacrim/al
nā zō lak′ ri məl

Lacrimal fluid is drained away by means of the

_____ / ___ / _____ / _____ duct.

1485

Lacrimal fluid keeps the surface of the eye moistened. It is continually forming and being removed. When there is more formed than can be removed by the apparatus, you say the person is

crying or tearing

_____.

1486

Lacrimation means crying. Excessive lacrimation is called **dacry**orrhea. This word gives you another word root for **tear.** It is _____.

dacry

1487

Look up words beginning with dacry in your medical dictionary. The combining form of the word root **dacry** is ___ cry / ___ .

dacry/o

1488

Analyze (you draw the diagonals):
dacryocystitis

_____

dacryoadenalgia

_____

dacryoma

_____

dacry/o/cyst/itis
dak rē ō sis tī′ tis

dacry/o/aden/algia
dak rē ō ad ə nal′ jē ə

dacry/oma
dak rē ō′ mə

1489

Analyze:
dacryopyorrhea

_____

dacryocystocele

_____

dacryolith

_____

dacry/o/py/orrhea

dacry/o/cyst/o/cele

dacry/o/lith
(You pronounce)

1490

If necessary you may use your dictionary to complete the following:
Dacryorrhea means

** _____.

Dacryocystoptosis means

** _____.

excessive flow of tears

prolapse of the tear sac

answer column	
instrument for cutting (incising) the tear sac (your own words, of course)	A dacryocystotome is ** _____. See "Case Study: Ophthalmology Report" on opposite page.
the ingestion (destruction or eating) of cells by phagocytes	**1491** Cyt/o/phag/o/cyt/osis is ** _____ _____.
the ingestion of cells by phagocytes	**1492** Cyt/o/phag/y is another way of saying ** _____ _____.
cyt/o/meter sī tom′ ə tər cyt/o/metry sī tom′ ə trē	**1493** An instrument for measuring cells is a _____ / _____ / _____. The process of measuring cells is _____ / ____ / _____.
cyt/o/stasis sī tos′ tə sis cyt/o/scop/y sī tos′ kə pē	**1494** Stopping or controlling cells is called _____ / ____ / _____. Examination of cells is _____ / ____ / _____ / ___.
nails	**1495** Look in your dictionary for words beginning with onych. These words refer to the _____.
onych/o	**1496** By studying words beginning with onych, you can find its combining form. The word root–combining form that refers to **nail** is _____ / ___.

onych/oid
on′ i koid
 	
onych/oma
on i kō′ mə
onych/osis
on i kō′ sis
	1497
	Build a word meaning:
	   resembling a fingernail
	       _____ / _____;
	
	   tumor of the nail (or nail bed)
	       _____;
	
	   any nail condition
	       _____.

246

CASE STUDY: OPHTHALMOLOGY REPORT

DIAGNOSIS: Intermittent alternating divergent strabismus (esophoria).

PROCEDURE: Bilateral lateral rectus recession 5–6 mm.

SURGICAL PROCEDURE: The eyes were prepped in the usual manner. The left eye was done first. A black 6–0 silk suture was placed at the lateral limbus and the eye rotated medially. A conjunctival incision was made over the insertion of the lateral rectus muscle, which was placed on a Prinz forceps and severed from its attachment to the globe. The intermuscular membrane check ligaments were cut and the muscles recessed 5–6 mm on the sclera with two 6–0 Chromic catgut sutures. The conjunctiva was closed with a running 6–0 Chromic catgut suture. The right eye was done in a similar procedure. A black, silk 6–0 suture was placed through the lateral limbus, the eye rotated medially, and a conjunctival incision made over the insertion of the lateral rectus muscle and Tenon's capsule buttonholed above and below it. The muscle was placed on a Prinz forceps, severed from its attachments to the globe, and recessed 5–6 mm on the sclera with two 6–0 Chromic catgut sutures after cutting the intramuscular membrane and the check ligaments. The conjunctiva was closed with a running 6–0 Chromic catgut suture. Acromycin Ophthalmic Ointment was instilled in the eyes, and patch and shields were applied. The patient was discharged to the recovery room in good condition.

---

answer column	
	1498
	Build a word meaning:
	softening of the nails
onych/o/malac/ia	_____ / / _____ / ____ ;
	fungus infection (condition) of the nails
onych/o/myc/osis	_____ / / _____ / ____ ;
onych/o/phag/ia (You pronounce)	nail biting (eating)
	_____ / / _____ / ____ .
hidden nail or condition of nail being hidden	**1499**
	Onych/o/crypt/osis means literally ** _____ _____ .
	1500
	Look up onychocryptosis in your dictionary. It refers to an
ingrown toenail	* _____ .
	~~1501~~
hair	**trich/o** is used in words to mean hair. A trich/o/ genous substance promotes the growth of _____ .

247

1502
Lith/iasis is the formation of calculi (in the wrong place). Trich/iasis is the formation of _____ (in the wrong places).

1503
Using trich/o, build a word meaning:
  hairy heart (noun)

  _____ / ___ / ___ / ___ ;

  hairy tongue (noun)

  _____ / ___ / ___ / ___ ;

  resembling hair

  _____ / ___ ;

  abnormal fear of hair

  _____ / ___ / ___ / ___ ;

  any hair disease

  _____ / ___ / ___ / ___ .

trichocardia
trik ō kār′ dē ə

trichoglossia
trik ō glos′ ē ə

trichoid

trichophobia

trichopathy

1504
phag/o means _____ . (You may refer to Frame 526 if necessary.)

1505
A phag/o/cyt/e is a cell that _____ micro-organisms. Phag/o/cyt/osis is the process of the cells _____ microorganisms.

1506
A large phagocyte is called a macr/o/phag/e. A small phagocyte is called a

  _____ / ___ / ___ / ___ .

micr/o/phag/e
microphage
mī′ krō fāj

1507
Onych/o/phag/y is nail biting. A word that means hair swallowing is

  _____ / ___ / ___ / ___ .

Air swallowing is

  _____ / ___ / ___ / ___ .

To understand and recognize suffixes, use the following chart to work Frames 1508 through 1524.

NOUN SUFFIXES	ORDINARY EXAMPLES
ism—condition, state, or theory	communism
tion—condition or action	stimulation satisfaction
ist ⎫ er ⎭ —one who ity—quality	communist prompter readability
ADJECTIVAL SUFFIXES	
ous—condition, material	pious porous
able ⎫ ible ⎭ —ability	readable edible

answer column

condition or state

1508
Crypt/orchid/ism is the _____ of having undescended testes.

condition or state

condition or state

1509
Hyper/thyroid/ism is a _____ of too much secretion by the thyroid gland. Iso/dactyl/ism is a _____ involving fingers of equal length.

theory

1510
Darwin/ism presents a theory of development. Mendel/ism presents a _____ of heredity.

noun

1511
Hypo/pituitar/ism is a _____ (noun/adjective).

action

1512
Contraction is the _____ of short-ening muscles.

condition

1513
Relaxation is a _____ of diminished tension.

nouns

1514
Contraction and relaxation are_____.
(nouns/adjectives)

249

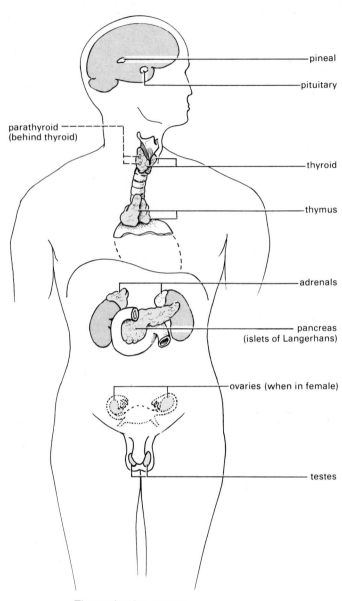

The endocrine system

labels:
- pineal
- pituitary
- parathyroid (behind thyroid)
- thyroid
- thymus
- adrenals
- pancreas (islets of Langerhans)
- ovaries (when in female)
- testes

answer column

---

one who

one who

1515

A psychiatrist is *_____ practices psychiatry. A medical practitioner is
*_____ practices medicine.

---

noun

1516

The word practitioner is a _____.

(noun/adjective)

1517

quality

Conductivity expresses the _____ of nervous tissue related to transferring impluses.

quality

Sensitivity expresses the _____ of nervous tissue related to receiving stimuli.

1518

noun

Irritability is a _____ .

(noun/adjective)

1519

material

Mucous refers to the nature of a _____ secreted by the mucous membrane. Serous refers

material

to the nature of the _____ lining body cavities.

1520

condition

Nervous refers to the _____ of being under too much tension.

1521

adjectives

Words ending in **ous** are _____ .

(nouns/adjectives)

1522

To say a food is digestible is to say it has the

ability

_____ to be digested. To say a fracture is

ability

reducible is to say that it has the _____ to be set.

1523

To say that lungs are inflatable is to say that they

ability

have the _____ to inflate.

1524

adjectives

Words ending in **ible** or **able** are _____ .

(nouns/adjectives)

1525

emia is a suffix that you have used without a formal introduction. If you understand emia thoroughly (which will show by your answer in Frame 1526, you may skip Frames 1527 and 1528.

251

answer column

condition of blood or blood condition	**1526** **emia** is a suffix that means *_____ _____.
leuk/emia leukemia lōō kē′ mē ə	**1527** Isch/emia is a condition in which blood is drained from one place. Blood cancer (too many leuk/o/cytes in the blood) is called _____/_____.
an/emia ə nē′ mē ə hyper/emia hī pər ē′ mē ə ur/emia yoo rē′ mē ə	**1528** Build a word meaning: without (not enough) blood _____/_____; too much blood (in one part) _____/_____; urine constituents in blood _____/_____.
see introduction	**1529** You now know a good system for word building.
see review sheets in Appendix A.	**1530** You know many prefixes, suffixes, and combining forms. You even know how to find word root–combining forms from singular and plural forms of a word.
intermittently for the last 167 frames	**1531** You also know several ways to find combining forms in your dictionary.
a wound or injury	**1532** To prove it again, look up trauma in your dictionary. It means a *_____.
traumat/o	**1533** Look at the next several words following trauma. The combining form for trauma is _____/_____.

252

1534

The study of caring for wounds is called

_____ / / _____ / ___.

Work Review Sheets 41 and 42

Each of these medical specialties uses medical terminology. Using your knowledge of word-building systems, complete the following chart. Check your answers on page 254.

SPECIALTY	SPECIALIST	LIMITS OF FIELD
pathology	1536	diseases—nature and causes
1537	dermatologist	1538
neurology	1539	nervous system diseases
1540	gynecologist	female diseases
urology	1541	male diseases and all urinary diseases
1542	end/o/crin/o/log/ist	glands of internal secretion
oncology	1543	neoplasms (new growths)
1544	1545	heart
ophthalmology	1546	eye
1547–1549	otorhinolaryngologist	1535
obstetrics	1548	pregnancy, childbirth, and puerperium
1549	geriatrician	old age
pediatrics	1550	children
orthopedics	orthopedist .	bones and muscles
psychiatry	1551	mental disorders

Check your answers on the next page.

SPECIALTY	SPECIALIST	LIMITS OF FIELD
	pathologist	
dermatology		skin
	neurologist	
gynecology		
	urologist	
endocrinology		
	oncologist	
cardiology	cardiologist	
	ophthalmologist	
otorhinolaryngology		ear−nose−throat

	obstetrician	
geriatrics		
	pediatrician	

	pyschiatrist	

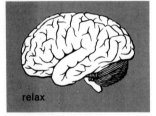

relax

1552
See, you really are competent in systematic medical terminology.

Congratulations on your completion of this programmed text in **medical terminology.** For further competence in medical communication, read and study the medical terminology review sheets in Appendix A. Then learn the extra medical word parts in Appendix C. Finally, learn the correct medical abbreviations and their meanings in Appendix D.

254

APPENDIX A
REVIEW SHEETS

(pain) in the liver and
Kidney

hepato/nephalgia

REVIEW SHEET
Number 1
FRAMES 95 TO 225

Following are a series of review sheets. Whenever a form is beginning to fade in your memory, you should rework the previous review sheets. Work them often. Cover the right column with a piece of paper and move it down as you do each word part.

WORD PART	MEANING	
acr/o	_____	extremity
megal/o	_____	enlargement
dermat/o	_____	skin
cyan/o	_____	blue
derm/o	_____	skin
leuk/o	_____	white
penia	_____	lack of
cardi/o	_____	heart
gastr/o	_____	stomach
cyt/o	_____	cell
algia	_____	pain
ectomy	_____	excision
otomy	_____	incision
ostomy	_____	new opening
duoden/o	_____	duodenum
electr/o	_____	electricity
tome	_____	cutting instrument
emia	_____	in the blood
chlor/o	_____	green
xanth/o	_____	yellow
erythr/o	_____	red

257

melan/o	_____	black
thromb/o	_____	clot
blast	_____	embryonic cell
paralysis	_____	loss of movement

REVIEW SHEET
Number 2
FRAMES 95 TO 225

Cover the right column with a sheet of paper and move it down as you finish each word part. A word part may be a word root, combining form, prefix, or suffix.

MEANING	WORD PART	
cutting instrument	_____	tome
in the blood	_____	emia
green	_____	chlor/o
enlargement	_____	megal/o
electricity	_____	electr/o
white	_____	leuk/o
yellow	_____	xanth/o
incision	_____	**ot**omy
blue	_____	cyan/o
red	_____	erythr/o
stomach	_____	gastr/o
extremity	_____	acr/o
black	_____	melan/o
new opening	_____	**os**tomy
skin	_____	dermat/o–derm/o
heart	_____	cardi/o
skin	_____	derm/o–dermat/o
clot	_____	thromb/o
embryonic cell	_____	blast
excision	_____	**ec**tomy
lack of	_____	penia
duodenum	_____	duoden/o

259

pain	_____	algia
cell	_____	cyt/o
loss of movement	_____	paralysis

REVIEW SHEET
Number 3
FRAMES 226 TO 330

Cover the right column with a sheet of paper and move it down as you finish each word part.

WORD PART	MEANING	
mania	_____	madness
hyper	_____	more than normal (above)
hypo	_____	less than normal (below)
emesis	_____	vomiting
throph/o	_____	development
aden/o	_____	gland
path/o	_____	disease
lip/o	_____	fat
encephal/o	_____	brain
oma	_____	tumor
cerebr/o	_____	cerebrum (brain)
crani/o	_____	cranium (skull)
mening/o	_____	meninges
carcin/o	_____	cancer
malac/o	_____	softening
muc/o	_____	mucus
cephal/o	_____	head
dynia	_____	pain
cele	_____	herniation
gram	_____	record

REVIEW SHEET
Number 4
FRAMES 226 TO 330

X

MEANING	WORD PART	
tumor	_____	oma
cerebrum (brain)	_____	cerebr/o
cranium (skull)	_____	crani/o
meninges	_____	mening/o
cancer	_____	carcin/o
softening	_____	malac/o
mucus	_____	muc/o
head	_____	cephal/o
pain	_____	dynia
record	_____	gram
brain	_____	encephal/o
fat	_____	lip/o
disease	_____	path/o
gland	_____	aden/o
development	_____	throph/o
vomiting	_____	emesis
less than normal (below)	_____	hypo
more than normal (above)	_____	hyper
madness	_____	mania
herniation	_____	cele

263

REVIEW SHEET
Number 5
FRAMES 331 TO 402

X

WORD PART	MEANING	
ten/o	_____	tendon
scope	_____	looking instrument
scopy	_____	looking procedure
burs/o	_____	bursa (serous sac)
inter	_____	between
abdomin/o	_____	abdomen
hydro	_____	water
phobia	_____	fear
oste/o	_____	bone
arthr/o	_____	joint
chondr/o	_____	cartilage
cost/o	_____	rib
inter	_____	between
dent/o	_____	tooth
ab	_____	from
ad	_____	toward
abdomin/o	_____	abdomen ✓
cyst/o	_____	bladder
centesis	_____	puncture
thorac/o	_____	thorax or chest
hydr/o	_____	water ✓
therap/o	_____	treatment
pub/o	_____	pubis
metr/o, meter	_____	measure
pelv/i	_____	pelvis

REVIEW SHEET
Number 6
FRAMES 331 TO 402

X

MEANING	WORD PART	
thorax or chest	_____	thorac/o
puncture	_____	centesis
bladder	_____	cyst/o
abdomen	_____	abdomin/o
toward	_____	ad
from	_____	ab
tooth	_____	dent/o
between	_____	inter
rib	_____	cost/o
cartilage	_____	chondr/o
joint	_____	arthr/o
bone	_____	oste/o
pelvis	_____	pelv/i
water	_____	hydr/o
treatment	_____	therap/o
pubis	_____	pub/o
measure	_____	metr/o, meter
fear	_____	phobia
water	_____	hydro
abdomen	_____	abdomin/o
between	_____	inter
bursa (serous sac)	_____	burs/o
looking procedure	_____	scopy
looking instrument	_____	scope
tendon	_____	ten/o

267

REVIEW SHEET
Number 7
FRAMES 403 TO 456

Suffixes that make a word an adjective meaning pertaining to:

SUFFIXES	EXAMPLE
al	duoden/al
ic	gastr/ic
ar	palm/ar
ac	cardi/ac

Prepare a list of word roots taking **al** and word roots taking **ic** to make them adjectives. Add to this list as you progress through your course.

al	ic	ar	ac

269

REVIEW SHEET
Number 8
FRAMES 457 TO 561

WORD PART	MEANING	
staphyl/o	uvula	uvula or staphylococcus
cocc/o	coccus	coccus
py/o	pus	pus
gen/o gen/ic	gen	generation
gen/esis	orig	origin
gen/ous	beg	beginning
orrhea	flow	flow
ot/o	ear	ear
rhin/o	nose	nose
lith/o	stone	stone or calculus
chol/e	gall	gall—bile
brad/y	low	slow
phag/o /ia	eat	eat
kinesi/o	movement	movement
log/o—logy —logist	study	study
malac/o	soften	softening
tach/y	rapid	fast
pne/o	breathe	breathe
a	without	without
dys	p.t.d.	bad, painful, difficult
peps/ia	digest	digestion
cyst/o	bladder	bladder
strept/o	twisted	twisted

271

dipl/o	*diplo*	double
uvul/o	*staphlo*	uvula
tympan/o	*ear drum*	ear drum

REVIEW SHEET
Number 9
FRAMES 457 TO 561

MEANING	WORD PART	
uvula	uvul/o	uvul/o
eardrum	tympan/o	tympan/o
double	dipl/o	dipl/o
flow	orrhea	orrhea
slow	brady	brad/y
digestion	pepsia	peps/ia
twisted	strept/o	strept/o
gall—bile	chole/o	chol/e
nose	rhino	rhin/o
pus	py/o	py/o
movement	kinesi/o	kinesi/o
fast	tachy	tach/y
beginning	acious	gen/ous—gen/o
origin	genesis	gen/esis
generation	genic	gen/ic
bad, painful, difficult	dys	dys
coccus	cocc/o	cocc/o
without	a	a
study	logo	log/o—logy—logist
stone or calculus	litho	lith/o
eat	phag/o	phag/o
uvula or staphylococcus	staphylo	staphyl/o
ear	ot/o	ot/o

273

breathe	*pne/o*	pne/o
bladder	*cyst/o*	cyst/o
softening	*malac/o*	malac/o

Rework previous review sheets.

REVIEW SHEET
Number 10
FRAMES 562 TO 653

WORD PART	MEANING	
neur/o	nerve	nerve
blast/o	emb form	embryonic form
angi/o	vessel	vessel
spasm	spasm	spasm
scler/o	hard	hard
my/o	muscle	muscle
fibr/o	fibrous	fibrous–fiber
lys/o	dest.	destruction
lip/o	fat	fat
cyt/o	cell	cell
hem/o	blood	blood
hemat/o	blood	blood
arthr/o	joint	joint
phob/o		fear
spermat/o	spermatozoa	spermatozoa
cyst/o	bladder	bladder
o/o		ovum
orchid/o	testicle	testicle
colp/o	vagina	vagina
metr/o	uterine tissue	uterine tissues
gynec/o	woman	woman
gen/o	origin	origin, beginning
oophor/o	ovary	ovary

275

pex/o /y	*fixation*	fixation
salping/o	*fallopia tube*	fallopian tube
hyster/o	*uterus*	uterus
cele	*hernia*	herniation
✓ ptosis	*prolapse*	prolapse

276

REVIEW SHEET
Number 11
Frames 562 to 653

MEANING	WORD PART	
woman	gynec/o	gynec/o
vagina	colop/o	co'
metr/o	ut tissue	uterine tissues
testicle	orchid	orchid/o
fear	phob/o	phob/o
vessel	angi/o	angi/o
uterus	hyster/o	hyster/o
destruction	lys/o	lys/o
origin, beginning	gen/o	gen/o
blood	hem/o	hemat/o–hem/o
blood	hemat/o	hem/o–hemat/o
bladder	cyst/o	cyst/o
hard	scler/o	scler/o
joint	arthr/o	arthr/o
fallopian tube	salping/o	salping/o
muscle	my/o	my/o
nerve	neur/o	neur/o
fixation	pex/y	pex/o
		/y
cell	cyt/o	cyt/o
embryonic form	blast/o	blast/o
ovary	oophor/o	oophor/o
herniation	cele	cele
disease	path/o	path/o

277

ovum	o/o	o/o
prolapse	ptosis	ptosis
fat	lip/o	lip/o
spermatozoa	spermat/o	spermat/o
fibrous–fiber	fibr/o	fibr/o
spasm	spasm	spasm

Rework previous review sheets.

REVIEW SHEET
Number 12
Frames 654 to 709

WORD PART	MEANING	
nephr/o	*kidney*	kidney
lith/o	*stone*	stone, calculus
pyel/o	*renal pelvis*	renal pelvis
plast/o /y	*surg. repair*	repair
ureter/o	*ureter*	ureter
ostomy	*new open*	new opening
orrhaphy	*suture*	suture
urethr/o	*urethra*	urethra
otomy	*incis.*	incision
ectomy	*excis*	excision
cyst/o	*bladder*	bladder
cyt/o	*cell*	cell
orrhagia	*hemm*	hemorrhage
orrhea	*flow*	flow
pneumon/o		lung
pneum/o	*air*	air
pne/o	*breathe*	breathing
melan/o	*black*	black
myc/o	*fungus*	fungus
carcin/o	*cancer*	cancer
rhin/o	*rhin/o*	nose
thorac/o	*thorax*	thorax or chest
meter, metr/o	*measure*	measure

279

ur/o	urine	urine
vesic/o	urinary bladder	urinary bladder
ren/o	kidney	kidney

REVIEW SHEET
Number 13
FRAMES 654 TO 709

MEANING	WORD PART	
hemorrhage	orrhagia	orrhagia ✓
cell	cyto	cyt/o
renal pelvis	pyel/o	pyel/o
measure	metro	meter–metr/o
urine	ur/o	ur/o
kidney	nethr/o	ren/o ✓
urinary bladder	✓ vesic/o	vesic/o
black	malan/o	melan/o
ureter	ureter/o	ureter/o
excision	ectomy	ectomy
kidney	ren/o	nephr/o
cancer	carcin/o	carcin/o
lung	pneumon/o	pneumon/o
urethra	urethr/o	urethr/o
thorax or chest	thorac/o	thorac/o
air	pneum/o	pneum/o
suture	orrhaphy	orrhaphy
nose	rhin/o	rhin/o
fungus	myc/o	myc/o
breathing	pne/o	pne/o
flow	orrhea	orrhea
bladder	cyst/o	cyst/o
incision	otomy	otomy

281

new opening	_ostomy_	ostomy
repair	_plasty_	plast/o
		/y
stone, calculus	_lith/o_	lith/o

Rework previous review sheets.

REVIEW SHEET
Number 14
FRAMES 710 to 761

WORD PART	MEANING	
stomat/o	mouth	mouth
dent/o	tooth	tooth
gloss/o	tongue	tongue
cheil/o	lips	lip
gingiv/o	gums	gum
esophag/o	esophagus	esophagus
gastr/o	stomach	stomach
enter/o	small int.	small intestine
duoden/o	colon duodenum	duodenum
col/o	rectum	colon
rect/o		rectum
proct/o	rectum an	anus or rectum
hepat/o	liver	liver
pancreat/o	pancreas	pancreas
clys/o,–clys/is	irr	wash–irrigate
ectas/ia, ectas/is	dialatestrtch	dilatation–stretch
scop/o	examine	examination
arteri/o	artery	artery
pleg/a /ia /ic	paralysis	paralysis
pex/o /y	fixation	fixation
hyster/o	uterus	uterus
orrhea	flow	flow

283

orrhaphy	_suture_	suture
cyst/o	_bladder_	bladder
splen/o	_spleen_	spleen

REVIEW SHEET
Number 15
FRAMES 710 TO 761

MEANING	WORD PART	
paralysis	*plegia*	pleg/a /ia /ic
duodenum	*duoden/o*	duoden/o
liver	*hepat/o*	hepat/o
suture	*orraphy*	orrhaphy
small intestine	*enter/o*	enter/o
spleen	*splen/o*	splen/o
tooth	*dent/o*	dent/o
flow	*orrhea*	orrhea
artery	*arteri/o*	arteri/o
anus or rectum	*proct/o*	proct/o
lip	*cheil/o*	cheil/o
wash—irrigate	*clys/o*	clys/is—clys/o
esophagus	*esophag/o*	esophag/o
uterus	*hyster/o*	hyster/o
bladder	*cyst/o*	cyst/o
fixation	*pex/o*	pex/o /y
examination	*scopo*	scop/o
colon	*col/o*	col/o
gum	*gingiv/o*	gingiv/o
mouth	*stomat/o*	stomat/o
dilatation—stretch	*ectasia*	ectas/ia /is

285

pancreas	_pancreat/o_	pancreat/o
rectum	_rect/o_	rect/o
tongue	_gloss/o_	gloss/o
stomach	_gastr/o_	gastr/o

Rework previous review sheets.

REVIEW SHEET
Number 16
FRAMES 762 TO 803

WORD PART	MEANING	
kinesi/o	movement	movement
arteri/o	artery	artery
orrhexis	rupture	rupture
orrhaphy	suture	suture
orrhea	flow	flow
orrhagia	hemorrhage	hemorrhage
esthesi/o	feeling	feeling–sensation
an–a	without	without
log/o	study	study
dys	bad difficult	bad, painful, difficult
hypo	under less	less than normal
par/a	around break	around–beyond
hyper	more than	more than normal
alges/i	oversens to pain	abnormal sensitivity
troph/o	develop	development
lys/o	dest	destruction
oste/o	bone	bone
arthr/o	joint	joint
phas/o	speech	speech
phon/o	voice	voice
tach/y	rapid	fast
brad/y	slow	slow
my/o	muscle	muscle
blast/o	embryonic	embryonic form

287

fibr/o	_fibrous_	fibrous, fiber
gram/o ✓	_recording_	recording
gram ✓	_record_	the record
graph ✓	_inst._	the instrument
graphy	_act process_	the process
phleb/o ✗	_vein_	vein

288

REVIEW SHEET
Number 17
FRAMES 762 TO 803

MEANING	WORD PART	
destruction	_lys/o_	lys/o
fast	_tach/y_	tach/y
flow	_orrhea_	orrhea
more than normal	_hyper_	hyper
fibrous, fiber	_fibr/o_	fibr/o
without	_an-a_	an–a
bone	_oste/o_	oste/o
joint	_arthr/o_	arthr/o
recording	_gram/o_	gram/o
the process	_graphy_	graphy
the instrument	_graph_	graph
the record	_____	gram
bad, painful, difficult	_dys_	dys
rupture	_orrhexia_	orrhexis
voice	_phon/o_	phon/o
muscle	_my/o_	my/o
feeling–sensation	_esthesi/o_	esthesi/o
less than normal	_hyp/o_	hypo
development	_troph/o_	troph/o
embryonic form	_blast/o_	blast/o
slow	_brady_	brad/y
suture	_orrhaphy_	orrhaphy
abnormal sensitivity	_algesi_	alges/i
study	_log/o_	log/o

289

artery		_arteri/o_	arteri/o
movement		_kinesi/o_	kinesi/o
around–beyond	✳	_par/a_	par/a
speech	⚹	_phas/o_	phas/o
hemorrhage	✳	_orrhagia_	orrhagia
vein	✳	_phleb/o_	phleb/o

Rework previous review sheets.

REVIEW SHEET
Number 18
FRAMES 804 TO 852

WORD PART	MEANING	
dipl/o	_double_	double
phon/o	_voice_	voice
opia	_vision_	vision
amb/i	_both_	both
cocc/o	_coccus_	coccus
cyan/o	_blue_	blue
neur/o	_nerve_	nerve
tripsy	_s. crushing_	surgical crushing
pyel/o	_renal pelvis_	renal pelvis
cyt/o	_cell_	cell
cyst/o	_bladder_	bladder
cele	_hernia_	herniation
dys	_bad pain_	bad, painful, difficult
chondr/o	_cart._	cartilage
cost/o	_rib_	rib
plas/o	_format._	formation, development
psych/o	_mind soul_	mind or soul
osis	_cond._	condition
oma	_tumor_	tumor
oid	_resemble_	resembling
pro	_before_	before
gnos/ia	_knowled_	knowledge or know
di/a	_through_	through
orrhea	_flow_	flow

291

orrhaphy	_suture_	suture
orrhagia	_hemmorage_	hemorrhage
orrhexis	_suture_	rupture
myel/o	_spine_	spinal cord
pharmac/o	_med. drugs_	drugs/medicine

292

REVIEW SHEET
Number 19
FRAMES 804 TO 852

MEANING	WORD PART	
drugs/medicine	*pharmaco*	pharmac/o
spinal cord	*myel/o*	myel/o
cell	*cyt/o*	cyt/o
formation, development	*plas/o*	plas/o
double	*dipl/o*	dipl/o
tumor	*oma*	oma
flow	*orrhea*	orrhea
blue	*cyan/o*	cyan/o
herniation	*cele*	cele
condition	*osis*	osis
rupture	*orrhexis*	orrhexis
coccus	*cocc/o*	cocc/o
renal pelvis	*pyel/o*	pyel/o
mind or soul	*psych/o*	psych/o
through	*di/a*	di/a
rib	*cost/o*	cost/o
hemorrhage	*orrhagia*	orrhagia
voice		phon/o
surgical crushing	*trips/y*	trips/y
suture	*orrhaphy*	orrhaphy
resembling	*oid*	oid
both	*amb/i*	amb/i
cartilage	*chondr/o*	chondr/o
before	*pro*	pro

293

vision	opia	opia
bad, painful, difficult	dys	dys
nerve	neur/o	neur/o
knowledge or know	gnos/ia	gnos/ia
bladder	cyst/o	cyst/o

REVIEW SHEET
Number 20
FRAMES 853 TO 888

WORD PART	MEANING	
therm/o	_heat_	heat
esthesi/o	_feeling_	feeling
metr/o, meter	_measure_	measure
phob/o	_fear_	fear
pleg/a	_paralysis_	paralysis
scop/o	_examine_	examine
micr/o	_small_	small
macr/o	_large_	large
cephal/o	_bone_	head
myel/o	_spine_	bone marrow
ot/o	_ear_	ear
rhin/o	_nose_	nose
cheil/o	_lips_	lip
dactyl/o	_finger toe_	finger or toe
megal/o	_enlarged_	enlargement
pol/y	_many_	many
ur/o	_urine_	urine
neur/o	_nerve_	nerve
psych/o	_mind soul_	mind or soul
arthr/o	_joint_	joint
oste/o	_bone_	bone
syn	_with_	with
drom/o	_sympt_	running with (symptom)
ectas/ia /is	_dilatation_	dilatation

REVIEW SHEET
Number 21
FRAMES 853 TO 888

MEANING	WORD PART	
bone marrow	myelo	myel/o
measure	metro	metr/o, meter
mind or soul	psycho	psych/o
nose	rhino	rhin/o
paralysis	plegia	pleg/ia
large	macro	macr/o
with	syn	syn
heat	therme	therm/o
finger or toe	dactylo	dactyl/o
urine	ur/o	ur/o
examine	scopo	scop/o
symptom	dromo	drom/o
enlargement	megal/o	megal/o
bone	osteo	oste/o
many	poly	pol/y
ear	oto	ot/o
joint	arthro	arthr/o
feeling	esthesio	esthesi/o
small	micro	micr/o
nerve	neuro	neur/o
lip	cheilo	cheil/o
head	cephalo	cephal/o
fear	phob	phob/o
dilatation	ectasia	ectas/ia /is

Rework previous review sheets.

297

REVIEW SHEET
Number 22
FRAMES 889 to 965

WORD PART	MEANING	
medi/o	middle	middle
later/o	side	side
omphal/o	umbilicus	umbilicus
bi/o	life living	living or life
lymph/o	lymph tissue	lymph tissue (fluid)
viscer/o	organ	organ
dips/o	thirst	thirst, drink
pol/y	many	many
mania	madness	madness
anter/o	in front of	before *in front*
poster/o	behind	behind, after
dors/o	back	back
ventr/o	belly	belly
cephal/o		head
encephal/o		brain
aer/o	air	air
chrom/o	color	color
lys/o	dest	destruction
metr/o meter	measure	measure
gen/o ic esis ous		beginning–formation
phil/o	att.	attraction
eu	easy	good
peps/ia	dig	digestion
kinesi/o	move	movement

men/o	*meneses*	menses–menstruation
stasis	*stophatt*	halt-control
syphil/o	*syphilus*	syphilis
pseud/o	*false*	false
edema	*swelling*	swelling
opia	*vision*	vision
ptosis	*prolapse*	prolapse
than/o	*death*	death
enter/o	*small intest*	small intestine

300

REVIEW SHEET
Number 23
FRAMES 889 TO 965

MEANING	WORD PART	
back	_____	dors/o
attraction	_____	phil/o
vision	_____	opia
madness	_____	mania
destruction	_____	lys/o
menses–menstruation	_____	men/o
swelling	_____	edema
measure	_____	metr/o, meter
thirst, drink	_____	dips/o
death	_____	than/o
middle	_____	medi/o
organ	_____	viscer/o
side	_____	later/o
lymph tissue (fluid)	_____	lymph/o
living or life	_____	bi/o
umbilicus	_____	omphal/o
small intestine	_____	enter/o
brain	_____	encephal/o
digestion	_____	peps/ia
syphilis	_____	syphil/o
prolapse	_____	ptosis
air	_____	aer/o
belly	_____	ventro/o
before	_____	anter/o

301

many	_____	pol/y
false	_____	pseud/o
halt–control	_____	stasis
movement	_____	kinesi/o
good	_____	eu
beginning–formation	_____	gen/o ic esis ous
color	_____	chrom/o
head	_____	cephal/o
behind–after	_____	poster/o

Rework previous review sheets.

REVIEW SHEET
Number 24
FRAMES 966 TO 987

WORD PART	MEANING	
lapar/o	_____	abdominal wall
hepat/o	_____	liver
col/o	_____	colon
bi/o	_____	life
pyr/o	_____	fever, fire
xanth/o	_____	yellow
chlor/o	_____	green
opia	_____	vision
erythr/o	_____	red
leuk/o	_____	white
melan/o	_____	black
cyt/o	_____	cell
cyst/o	_____	bladder
derm/o	_____	skin
blast/o	_____	embryonic form
emia	_____	blood
hidr/o	_____	sweat
aden/o	_____	gland
gynec/o	_____	woman
path/o	_____	disease
plast/o	_____	repair
ophthalm/o	_____	eye
viscer/o	_____	organ
glyc/o	_____	sugar
hypo	_____	less than normal
later/o	_____	side

REVIEW SHEET
Number 25
FRAMES 966 TO 987

MEANING	WORD PART	
gland	_____	aden/o
skin	_____	derm/o
white	_____	leuk/o
yellow	_____	xanth/o
disease	_____	path/o
bladder	_____	cyst/o
side	_____	later/o
organ	_____	viscer/o
sweat	_____	hidr/o
abdominal wall	_____	lapar/o
eye	_____	ophthalm/o
fever, fire	_____	pyr/o
less than normal	_____	hypo
embryonic form	_____	blast/o
liver	_____	hepat/o
woman	_____	gynec/o
black	_____	melan/o
sugar	_____	glyc/o
life	_____	bi/o
red	_____	erythr/o
blood	_____	emia
repair	_____	plast/o
colon	_____	col/o
green	_____	chlor/o
vision	_____	opia

Should you rework previous review sheets?

REVIEW SHEET
Number 26
FRAMES 988 TO 1038

WORD PART	MEANING	
mamm/o	breast	breast
stern/o	sternum	sternum
version	turning	turning
periton/o	peritonium	peritoneum
appendic/o	appendix	appendix
immun/o	immunity	immunity
dyn/o	pain	pain
spasm	spasm	spasm
orrhaphy	suture	suture
orrhea	flow	flow
orrhagia	hemm	hemorrhage
orrhexis	rupture	rupture
end/o	inner	inner
mes/o	middle	middle
ect/o	outer	outer
hyster/o	uterus	uterus
ectop/o ✓	misplaced	misplaced
retr/o	behind	behind–backward
par/a	around	around
hepat/o	liver	liver
aut/o	self	self
hem/o	blood	blood
py/o	pus	pus
muc/o	mucus	mucus

REVIEW SHEET
Number 27
FRAMES 988 TO 1038

MEANING	WORD PART	
outer–outside	_____	ect/o
pain	_____	dyn/o
rupture	_____	orrhexis
breast	_____	mamm/o
sternum	_____	stern/o
inner	_____	end/o
mucus	_____	muc/o
flow	_____	orrhea
behind–backward	_____	retr/o
turning	_____	version
peritoneum	_____	periton/o
blood	_____	hem/o
appendix	_____	appendic/o
middle	_____	mes/o
suture	_____	orrhaphy
immunity	_____	immun/o
uterus	_____	hyster/o
around	_____	par/a
pus	_____	py/o
liver	_____	hepat/o
misplaced	_____	ectop/o
hemorrhage	_____	orrhagia
spasm	_____	spasm

REVIEW SHEET
Number 28
FRAMES 1023 TO 1038

Count using these prefixes.

PREFIX	MEANING	
mono		single–one
multi		many
nulli		none
primi		first
uni		one
bi		two
diplo		double
tri		three
quad		four
quint		five
sex		six
septa		seven
octa		eight
nona		nine
deca		ten
centa		one hundred
kilo		one thousand

REVIEW SHEET
Number 29
FRAMES 1023 TO 1038

MEANING	PREFIX	
double	double	diplo
many	poly multi	multi
five	quint	quint
seven	septa	septa
one hundred	centa	centa
eight	octa	octa
two	bi	bi
nine	nona	nona
ten	deca	deca
single/one	mono	mono
first	primi	primi
one thousand	kilo	kilo
four	quad	quad
six	sex	sex
none	nulli	nulli
seven	septa	septa
three	tri	tri

REVIEW SHEET
Number 30
FRAMES 1039 TO 1120

WORD PART	MEANING	
par/o	_____	to bear
pyr/o	_____	heat or fire
ocul/o	_____	eye
or/o	_____	mouth
null/i	_____	none
ab	_____	from
ad	_____	toward
de	_____	from
ex	_____	from
narc/o	_____	sleep
leps/y	_____	seizure
is/o	_____	equal
anis/o	_____	unequal
dactyl/o	_____	fingers–toes
peri	_____	around
chondr/o	_____	cartilage
cost/o	_____	rib
aden/o	_____	gland
circum	_____	around
di/a	_____	through
per	_____	through
necr/o	_____	dead
ectomy	_____	excision
otomy	_____	incision

315

phob/o	_____	fear
phil/o	_____	attraction
ectop/o	_____	misplaced
phag/o	_____	eat

REVIEW SHEET
Number 31
FRAMES 1039 TO 1120

MEANING	WORD PART	
cartilage		chondr/o
sleep		narc/o
fingers–toes		dactyl/o
attraction		phil/o
from		de–ab–ex
from		ab–de–ex
from		ex–ab–de
heat or fire		pyr/o
mouth		or/o
eye		ocul/o
to bear		par/o
incision		otomy
rib		cost/o
toward		ad
excision		ectomy
fear		phob/o
none		null/i
seizure		leps/y
dead		necr/o
equal		is/o
gland		aden/o
through		per–di/a
through		di/a–per
misplaced		ectop/o

317

unequal	———————————	anis/o
around	———————————	circum–peri
around	———————————	peri–circum
eat	———————————	phag/o

Should you rework previous review sheets?

REVIEW SHEET
Number 32
FRAMES 1121 TO 1192

WORD PART	MEANING	
pod/o	————————————	foot
ren/o	————————————	kidney
a or an	————————————	without
meta	————————————	beyond
carp/o	————————————	carpals (wrist bones)
tars/o	————————————	tarsals (ankle bones)
stasis	————————————	control
hom/o	————————————	same
heter/o	————————————	different
lys/o	————————————	destruction
pex/o	————————————	fixation
sym	————————————	together
super	————————————	above
pub/o	————————————	pubis
supra	————————————	above
par/a	————————————	bear
syn	————————————	together
metr/o, hyster/o	————————————	uterus
orrhexis	————————————	rupture
orrhaphy	————————————	suture
salping/o	————————————	fallopian tube
oophor/o	————————————	ovary
epi	————————————	over–upon
extra	————————————	in addition to–beyond

319

infra	————————————	below–under
sub	————————————	under–below
sept/o	————————————	infection
phag/o	————————————	eat
anti	————————————	against
contra	————————————	against
trans	————————————	across–over
trips/y	————————————	crushing
ectop/o	————————————	misplaced

REVIEW SHEET
Number 33
FRAMES 1121 TO 1192

MEANING	WORD PART	
control	_____	stasis
tarsals (ankle bones)	_____	tars/o
carpals (wrist bones)	_____	carp/o
beyond	_____	meta
without	_____	a or an
kidney	_____	ren/o
foot	_____	pod/o
under–below	_____	sub
below–under	_____	infra
in addition to–beyond	_____	extra
over–upon	_____	epi
ovary	_____	oophor/o
fallopian tube	_____	salping/o
suture	_____	orrhaphy
rupture	_____	orrhexis
uterus	_____	metr/o, hyster/o
together	_____	syn
bear	_____	par/a
above	_____	supra
pubis	_____	pub/o
above	_____	super
together	_____	sym
fixation	_____	pex/o
destruction	_____	lys/o
different	_____	heter/o
same	_____	hom/o

REVIEW SHEET
Number 34
FRAMES 1193 to 1265

WORD PART	MEANING	
sept/o or seps/is	_____	infection
phag/o	_____	eat
anti	_____	against
contra	_____	against
trans	_____	across–over
trips/y	_____	crushing
ectop/o	_____	misplaced
vagin/o	_____	vagina
urethr/o	_____	urethra
in	_____	in or not
somn/i	_____	sleep
cis/e	_____	cut
mal	_____	bad
sanguin/o	_____	blood
natal	_____	birth
febrile	_____	fever
partum	_____	birth
tri	_____	three
bi	_____	two–double
semi	_____	half
hemi	_____	half
troph/o	_____	development
con	_____	with
dis	_____	to free–to undo

post	_____	after, behind
pre	_____	before, in front of
intra	_____	within

REVIEW SHEET
Number 35
FRAMES 1193 TO 1265

MEANING	WORD PART	
within	_____	intra
before, in front of	_____	pre
after, behind	_____	post
to free–to undo	_____	dis
with	_____	con
development	_____	troph/o
half	_____	hemi
half	_____	semi
two–double	_____	bi
three	_____	tri
cut	_____	cis/e
sleep	_____	somn/i
in or not	_____	in
urethra	_____	urethr/o
vagina	_____	vagin/o
birth	_____	partum
fever	_____	febrile
birth	_____	natal
blood	_____	sanguin/o
bad	_____	mal
misplaced	_____	ectop/o
crushing	_____	trips/y
across–over	_____	trans
against	_____	contra

against	_____	anti
eat	_____	phag/o
infection	_____	sept/o or seps/is

REVIEW SHEET
Number 36

Make plurals of these singular terms.

SINGULAR	PLURAL	
bursa	*ae*	bursae
conjunctiva	*ae*	conjunctivae
fossa	*ae*	fossae
vertebra	*ae*	vertebrae
pleura	*ae*	pleurae
cornea	*ae*	corneae
bacillus	*i*	bacilli
bronchus	*i*	bronchi
coccus	*i*	cocci
focus	*i*	foci
locus	*i*	loci
nucleus	*i*	nuclei
atrium	*a*	atria
ileum	*a*	ilea
bacterium	*a*	bacteria
carcinoma	*mata*	carcinomata
lipoma	*mata*	lipomata
condyloma	*mata*	condylomata
enema	*mata*	enemata
ganglion	*a*	ganglia
spermatozoon	*a*	spermatozoa
diagnosis	*es*	diagnoses
pelvis	*es*	pelves
appendix	*ices*	appendices
thorax	*aces*	thoraces
cervix	*ices*	cervices

327

REVIEW SHEET
Number 37
FRAMES 1266 TO 1349

WORD PART	MEANING	
phren/o	_____	diaphragm
ostomy	_____	permanent opening
lith/o	_____	stone
pleur/o	_____	pleural membrane
plegia	_____	paralysis
ped/o	_____	foot
man/o	_____	hand
pod/o	_____	foot
chir/o	_____	hand
hist/o	_____	tissue
cervic/o	_____	neck of uterus–neck
nas/o	_____	nose
pharyng/o	_____	pharynx
laryng/o	_____	larynx
trache/o	_____	trachea
bronch/o	_____	bronchus
pleur/o	_____	pleura
centesis	_____	puncture
sinistr/o	_____	left
dextr/o	_____	right
vas/o	_____	vessel
ne/o	_____	new
penia	_____	lack of
splen/o	_____	spleen
uni	_____	one

REVIEW SHEET
Number 38
FRAMES 1266 TO 1349

MEANING	WORD PART	
nose	_____	nas/o
pleura	_____	pleur/o
before, in front of	_____	pre
lack of	_____	penia
one	_____	uni
larynx	_____	laryng/o
puncture	_____	centesis
right	_____	dextr/o
bronchus	_____	bronch/o
vessel	_____	vas/o
spleen	_____	splen/o
three	_____	tri
left	_____	sinistr/o
trachea	_____	trache/o
new	_____	ne/o
pharynx	_____	pharyng/o
neck of uterus, neck	_____	cervic/o
tissue	_____	hist/o
hand	_____	chir/o
foot	_____	pod/o
hand	_____	man/o
foot	_____	ped/o
paralysis	_____	pleg/ia
pleural membrane	_____	pleur/o

331

stone	_____	lith/o
permanent opening	_____	ostomy
diaphragm	_____	phren/o

Rework previous review sheets.

REVIEW SHEET
Number 39
FRAMES 1350 TO 1428

WORD PART	MEANING	
noct/i	_____	night
nyct/o	_____	night
opia	_____	vision
ankyl/o	_____	stiff
phor/o	_____	bear—carry
eu	_____	good, well, easy
stasis	_____	stopping, controlling
calcane/o	_____	heel
carp/o	_____	wrist
schiz/o, schist/o, or schisis	_____	split
ischi/o	_____	ischium
stern/o	_____	sternum
phalang/o	_____	phalanges
acromi/o	_____	acromion
humer/o	_____	humerus
condyl/o	_____	condyle
gangli/o	_____	ganglia
thromb/o	_____	clot, thrombus
trich/o	_____	hair
orrhexis	_____	rupture
ectop/o	_____	misplaced
ante	_____	before, forward
plasm/o	_____	formation

(handwritten: "pass through" next to phor/o; "siton" next to ischi/o)

333

rachi/o, rach/i	_____	spine
lumb/o	_____	lumbar
uln/o	_____	ulnar
radi/o	_____	radius
scapul/o	_____	scapula
phren/o	_____	mind or diaphragm
enter/o	_____	small intestine
fung/i, myc/o	_____	fungus
gloss/o	_____	tongue
cheil/o	_____	lips

REVIEW SHEET
Number 40
FRAMES 1350 TO 1428

MEANING	WORD PART	
lips	_____	cheil/o
tongue	_____	gloss/o
fungus	_____	fung/i, myc/o
small intestine	_____	enter/o
mind or diaphragm	_____	phren/o
scapula	_____	scapul/o
radius	_____	radi/o
ulnar	_____	uln/o
lumbar	_____	lumb/o
spine	_____	rachi/o, rach/i
split	_____	schisis, schist/o, or schiz/o
bear, carry	_____	phor/o
night	_____	nyct/o–noct/i
night	_____	noct/i–nyct/o
before, forward	_____	ante
wrist	_____	carp/o
formation	_____	plasm/o, plas/o, troph/o, gen/o
clot, thrombus	_____	thromb/o
stopping, controlling	_____	stasis
hair	_____	trich/o
humerus	_____	humer/o

335

heel	_____	calcane/o
misplaced	_____	ectop/o
sternum	_____	stern/o
rupture	_____	orrhexis
ganglia	_____	gangli/o
ischium	_____	ischi/o
vision	_____	opia
condyle	_____	condyl/o
acromion	_____	acromi/o
good, well, easy	_____	eu
phalanges	_____	phalang/o
stiff	_____	ankyl/o

Rework previous review sheets.

REVIEW SHEET
Number 41
FRAMES 1429 to 1534

WORD PART	MEANING	
ophthal/mo	_____	eye
xanth/o	_____	yellow
chlor/o	_____	green
erythr/o	_____	red
blephar/o	_____	eyelid
py/o	_____	pus
phag/o	_____	ingesting
trich/o	_____	hair
traumat/o	_____	injury
onc/o	_____	neoplasms
corne/o	_____	cornea
scler/o	_____	sclera
ir/o	_____	iris
irid/o	_____	iris
retin/o	_____	retina
cor/e, core/o	_____	pupil
kerat/o	_____	cornea
cycl/o	_____	ciliary body
pleg/ia	_____	paralysis
lacrim/o	_____	tear
dacry/o	_____	tear
tome	_____	instrument for incising
tympan/o	_____	eardrum
ren/o	_____	kidney

vesic/o	_____	bladder
pod/o	_____	foot
chir/o	_____	hands
crypt/o	_____	hidden
emia	_____	blood
rachi/o, rach/i	_____	spine
omphal/o	_____	navel
onych/o	_____	nail
phren/o	_____	diaphragm
om/o	_____	shoulder
myx/o	_____	mucus

338

REVIEW SHEET
Number 42
FRAMES 1429 TO 1534

MEANING	WORD PART	
bladder	_____	vesic/o
cornea	_____	kerat/o–corne/o
cornea	_____	corne/o–kerat/o
blood	_____	emia
mucus	_____	myx/o–muc/o
instrument for incising	_____	tome
iris	_____	ir/o–irid/o
iris	_____	irid/o–ir/o
diaphragm	_____	phren/o
retina	_____	retin/o
tear	_____	dacry/o–lacrim/o
tear	_____	lacrim/o–dacry/o
nail	_____	onych/o
hands	_____	chir/o
eardrum	_____	tympan/o
shoulder	_____	om/o
navel	_____	omphal/o
ciliary body	_____	cycl/o
sclera	_____	scler/o
foot	_____	pod/o
neoplasms	_____	onc/o
injury	_____	traumat/o
hair	_____	trich/o
ingesting	_____	phag/o

pus	_____	py/o
eyelid	_____	blephar/o
red	_____	erythr/o
green	_____	chlor/o
yellow	_____	xanth/o
eye	_____	ophthal/mo
spine	_____	rachi/o, rach/i
hidden	_____	crypt/o
kidney	_____	ren/o
pupil	_____	cor/e, core/o
paralysis	_____	pleg/ia

You can rework review sheets anytime.

APPENDIX B
LIST OF WORD PARTS LEARNED

WORD PART	INTRODUCED IN FRAME NUMBER	WORD PART	INTRODUCED IN FRAME NUMBER
a	542	cardi/o	163
ab	403	carp/o	1391
abdomin/o	422	caud/o	905
acr/o	98	cele	294
acromi/o	1414	centesis	425
ad	414	cephal/o	279
aden/o	248	cerebr/o	313
aer/o	922	cervic/o	1282
alges/i	778	cheil/o	721
algia	189	chir/o	1328
amb/i	808	chlor/o	134
amni/o	427	chol/e	512
an	775	chondr/o	352
angi/o	563	chrom/o	934
anis/o	1079	circum	1090
ankyl/o	1363	clys/o	731
ante	1249	cocc/o	462
anter/o	897	col/o	734
anti	1175	colp/o	615
appendic/o	1275	con	1232
arteri/o	568	condyl/o	1420
arthr/o	339	contra	1181
aut/o	1015	cor/e, core/o	1468
bi	1216	corne/o	1450
bi/o	924	cortic/o	1276
blast/o	563	cost/o	357
blephar/o	1446	crani/o	306
brad/y	525	crypt/o	591
bronch/o	1286	cyan/o	115
burs/o	351	cycl/o	1476
calcane/o	1386	cyst/o	430
carcin/o	261	cyt/o	146

·(Continued)

WORD PART	INTRODUCED IN FRAME NUMBER
dacry/o	1486
dactyl/o	867
de	1045
dent/o	368
derm/o	133
dermat/o	110
dextr/o	1322
di/a	847
dipl/o	804
dips/o	890
dis	1242
dors/o	901
drom/o	881
duoden/o	199
dyn/ia	283
dys	553
ect/o	990
ectas/ia, ectas/is	729
ectomy	193
ectop/o	1002
edema	960
electr/o	184
emesis	242
emia	138
encephal/o	292
end/o	988
enter/o	729
epi	1145
erythr/o	134
esophag/o	759
esthesi/o	775
eu	940
ex	1057
external	898
extra	1150
femor/o	1404
fibr/o	566
gangli/o	1423
gastr/o	168
gen/o	484
gingiv/o	725
gloss/o	716
glyc/o	980

WORD PART	INTRODUCED IN FRAME NUMBER
gnos/ia	842
gram/o	185
graph/o	186
gynec/o	651
hem/o	572
hemat/o	574
hemi	1227
hepat/o	747
heter/o	1126
hidr/o	975
hist/o	1340
hom/o	1121
humer/o	1416
hydr/o	445
hyper	232
hypo	233
hyster/o	631
iasis	514
iatr	1327
in	1197
infra	1155
inter	363
intr/a	1261
ir/o	1452
irid/o	1460
is/o	1073
ischi/o	1397
itis	114
kerat/o	1473
kinesi/o	796
lacrim/o	1480
lapar/o	966
laryng/o	1296
later/o	897
leps/y	1069
leuk/o	134
lip/o	259
lith/o	508
log/o	180
lumb/o	376
lymph/o	954
lys/o	567
macr/o	863

(Continued)

WORD PART	INTRODUCED IN FRAME NUMBER	WORD PART	INTRODUCED IN FRAME NUMBER
mal	1209	oste/o	331
malac/o	300	ostomy	201
mania	173	ot/o	491
medi/o	897	otomy	207
megal/o	104	pancreat/o	751
melan/o	134	par/a	781
men/o	553	paralysis	121
mening/o	326	par/o	1031
mes/o	989	path/o	255
meta	1164	pelv/i	393
metr/o, meter	400	penia	151
metr/o (uterus)	635	peps/o	557
micr/o	859	per	1100
mon/o	1023	peri	1086
muc/o	269	pex/o	605
mult/i	1027	phag/o	526
my/o	789	phalang/o	1411
myc/o	696	pharmac/o	841
myel/o	822	pharyng/o	1286
narc/o	1064	phas/o	784
nas/o	1286	phil/o	1115
ne/o	1344	phleb/o	763
necr/o	1107	phob/o	450
nephr/o	654	phon/o	786
nerv	60	phor/o	1369
neur/o	563	phren/o	1380
noct/i	1350	plas/o	825
null/i	1035	plasm/o	1345
nyct/o	1355	plast/o	345
o/o	597	pleg/o	1463
oid	266	pleur/o	1286
oma	252	pne/o	535
omphal/o	914	pneum/o	702
onych/o	1495	pneumon/o	681
oophor/o	600	pod/o	1326
ophthalm/o	1437	pol/y	871
opia	805	post	1247
orchid/o	588	poster/o	906
orrhagia	672	pre	1248
orrhaphy	665	prim/i	1036
orrhea	487	pro	844
orrhexis	767	proct/o	743
osis	119	pseud/o	958

(Continued)

WORD PART	INTRODUCED IN FRAME NUMBER	WORD PART	INTRODUCED IN FRAME NUMBER
psych/o	830	sub	1158
ptosis	644	super	897
pub/o	385	supra	380
py/o	478	sym	1131
pyel/o	659	syn	875
pyr/o	971	syphil/o	955
rach/i, rachi/o	1431	tach/y	530
rect/o	738	ten/o	355
ren/o	676	therap/o	455
retin/o	1465	therm/o	853
retr/o	1007	thorac/o	437
rhin/o	501	thromb/o	159
salping/o	610	tom	129
sanguin/o	1238	trache/o	1286
scapul/o	1413	trans	1188
schiz/o	1380	tri	1215
scler/o	565	trich/o	1501
scop/o	710	trips/y	819
semi	1227	troph/o	235
sept/o	1170	tympan/o	498
sinistr/o	1317	uni	1217
spasm	564	ur/o	658
spermat/o	582	ureter/o	662
spir/o	1195	urethr/o	669
splen/o	755	uvul/o	477
spondyl/o	1431	vas/o	1334
staphyl/o	468	ventr/o	908
stasis	952	vesic/o	675
stern/o	1406	viscer/o	962
stomat/o	711	xanth/o	134
strept/o	466		

APPENDIX C
ADDITIONAL WORD PARTS

Following are some word parts that you can use with your word-building system. (There are others, of course, but these build fairly important and useful words.) If you want to enlarge your vocabulary dramatically:

1. pick a word part that interests you,
2. look for it in your dictionary,
3. note how many words begin with this part,
4. list five of them with their meanings.

Other words that contain the word part you worked with exist; for example, **therm**/o/meter and hyper/**therm**/ia.

WORD PART	MEANING	EXAMPLE
acu	a needle	acupressure
actin/o	ray	actin/o/dermat/itis
all/o	other, different	all/o/plas/ia
ambl/y	dim, dull	ambl/y/op/ia
andr/o	man, male	andr/o/path/y
antr/o	cavity, antrum	antr/o/scop/y
atel/o	incomplete, imperfect	atel/o/gloss/ia
ather/o	porridge-like	ather/o/scler/osis
audi/o	hear, hearing	audi/o/meter
balan/o	glans (penis or clitoris)	balan/o/plast/y
bar/o	weight, heavy	hyp/o/bar/o/path/y
bil/i	bile	bil/i/ur/ia
brachi/o	upper arm	brachialgia
cac/o	bad, diseased, abnormal	cac/o/rhin/ia
cari/o	decay	cari/o/gen/ic
cat/a	down, downward	cat/a/leps/y
celi/o	abdominal region	celi/o/my/algia
cer	wax	cerosis
chron/o	time	chron/ic
clas/ia	breaking	arthr/o/clas/ia
cleis/is	closure, occlusion	colp/o/cleis/is
coll/o	glutinous, jellylike	coll/oid
copr/o	feces, excrement	copr/o/stas/is
prot/o	first	prot/o/plasm
pteryg/o	wing	pteryg/oid

(Continued)

WORD PART	MEANING	EXAMPLE
ptyal/o	saliva	ptyalogram
radicul/o	root	radicul/o/neur/itis
sarc/o	flesh	sarc/oma
scoli/o	curved, curvature	scoli/osis
scot/o	darkness	scot/oma
seb/o	sebum	seb/orrhea
sial/o	saliva	sial/o/aden/itis
sit/o	food	sit/o/therap/y
somat/o	body	psych/o/somat/ic
somn/o	sleep	in/somn/ia
son/o	sound	sonometer
sphygm/o	pulse	sphygm/o/man/o/meter
sten/o	narrowness, constriction	sten/osis
stere/o	solid, solid body	stere/o/gnos/is
steth/o	chest	steth/o/scop/e
sthen/o	strength	a/sthen/ia
stigmat/o	mark, point	a/stigmat/ism
tel/e	distant, far	tel/e/metr/y
terat/o	monster, wonder	terat/oma
tetr/a	four	tetr/a/log/y
thanat/o	death	thanat/oid
thel/o	nipple	thelorrhagia
trop/o	turning	heter/o/trop/ia
ultra	beyond	ultrasonic
varic/o	varicose vein	varic/o/cele
ven/o	vein, vena cava	ven/o/clys/is
xen/o	strange, foreign	xen/o/phob/ia
xer/o	dry	xer/o/derm/a

APPENDIX D
ABBREVIATIONS

The following lists of abbreviations are grouped by topic. They are arranged in columns to assist you in learning. Column 1 lists the abbreviation, column 2 lists the meaning, and column 3 is left blank as a work space. Study the abbreviation and its meaning. Then cover the abbreviation and read the meaning. Write the abbreviation correctly in the blank. You may use the same method to learn the meanings by covering the meaning and reading the abbreviation. Write the meaning correctly on a separate piece of paper.

WEIGHTS AND MEASURES

Metric:

kg	kilogram(s)	(1000 g)	_____
hg	hectogram	(100 g)	_____
dag	decagram	(10 g)	_____
g or gm	gram		_____
dg	decigram	(0.1 g)	_____
cg	centigram	(0.01 g)	_____
mg	milligram	(0.001 g)	_____
μg or mcg	microgram	(0.001 mg)	_____

Standard:

lb, #	pound	_____
oz, symbol	ounce	_____
dr, symbol	dram	_____
gr	grain	_____

Volume:

cumm	cubic millimeter	(mm^3)	_____
cc	cubic centimeter	(cm^3)	_____
cum	cubic meter	(m^3)	_____
cu in	cubic inch	(in^3)	_____
cu ft	cubic foot	(ft^3)	_____
cu yd	cubic yard	(yd^3)	_____

Lengths:

in, "	inch	(2.54 cm)	_____
ft, '	foot	(12 in)	_____
yd	yard	(36 in)	_____
mm	millimeter	(0.001 m)	_____
cm	centimeter	(0.01 m)	_____
m	meter		_____
km	kilometer	(1000 m)	_____

(Continued)

WEIGHTS AND MEASURES

Liquid Volume:

t, tsp	teaspoon		_____
T, Tbsp	tablespoon		_____
c	cup		_____
m, min	minims		_____
ml	milliliter	(0.001 L)	_____
cc	cubic centimeter	(1 ml)	_____
cl	centiliter	(0.01 L)	_____
dl	deciliter	(0.1 L)	_____
L	liter	(1000 ml)	_____
dal	decaliter	(10 L)	_____
hl	hectoliter	(100 L)	_____
kl	kiloliter	(1000 L)	_____
fl dr	fluid dram	(60 min)	_____
fl oz	fluid ounce	(8 fl dr)	_____
pt	pint	(16 oz)	_____
qt	quart	(32 oz)	_____
gal	gallon	(4 qt)	_____
gt	drop	(1 min)	_____
gtt	drops		_____

Miscellaneous:

at wt	atomic weight	_____
C, kcal	calorie	_____
c	curie	_____
ht	height	_____
mA	milliampere	_____
mEq	milliequivalent	_____
mHz	megahertz	_____
mg%	milligram percent	_____
mw	molecular weight	_____
IU	international units	_____
U	units	_____

CHEMICAL

Symbols:

Al	aluminum	_____
Ar	argon	_____
As	arsenic	_____
Ba	barium	_____
B	boron	_____
Br	bromine	_____
Cd	cadmium	_____
Ca	calcium [Ca^{2+} ion]	_____

(Continued)

348

CHEMICAL

C	carbon	_____
CO_2	carbon dioxide	_____
Cl	chlorine [Cl^- ion]	_____
Cr	chromium	_____
Co	cobalt	_____
Cu	copper [Cu^{2+} ion]	_____
F	fluorine	_____
$C_6H_{12}O_6$	glucose	_____
He	helium	_____
H	hydrogen	_____
I	iodine [^{131}I radioactive]	_____
Fe	iron	_____
Kr	krypton	_____
Pb	lead	_____
Li	lithium	_____
Mg	magnesium	_____
Mn	manganese	_____
Hg	mercury	_____
Ne	neon	_____
N	nitrogen	_____
O	oxygen (O_2)	_____
P	phosphorus	_____
K	potassium	_____
Ra	radium	_____
Se	selenium	_____
Si	silicon	_____
Ag	silver	_____
$AgNO_3$	silver nitrate	_____
Na	sodium	_____
NaCl	sodium chloride	_____
S	sulfur	_____
U	uranium	_____
Zn	zinc	_____

DIAGNOSES

ABE	acute bacterial endocarditis	_____
ACVD	acute cardiovascular disease	_____
AF (Afib)	atrial fibrillation	_____
AI	aortic insufficiency	_____
AID	acute infectious disease	_____
	artificial insemination donor	_____
AIDS	acquired immune deficiency syndrome	_____
AIH	artificial insemination husband	_____

349

(Continued)

DIAGNOSES

ALL	acute lymphocytic leukemia	_____
ALS	amyotrophic lateral scoliosis	_____
AMI	acute myocardial infarction	_____
AOD	arterial occlusive disease	_____
ARC	AIDS Related Complex (Conditions)	_____
ARD	acute respiratory disease	_____
ARF	acute respiratory failure	_____
	acute renal failure	_____
	acute rheumatic fever	_____
ARV	AIDS Related Virus	_____
AS	aortic stenosis	_____
	arteriosclerosis	_____
	left ear (auris sinistra)	_____
ASCVD	arteriosclerotic cardiovascular disease	_____
ASHD	arteriosclerotic heart disease	_____
BCC	basal cell carcinoma	_____
BO	body odor	_____
Ca	cancer	_____
CAD	coronary artery disease	_____
CHD	congestive heart disease	_____
	congenital hip dislocation	_____
CE	cardiac enlargement	_____
CF	cystic fibrosis	_____
CHD	congenital or coronary heart disease	_____
	childhood disease	_____
CHF	congestive heart failure	_____
CIS	carcinoma in situ	_____
CLD	chronic liver disease	_____
	chronic lung disease	_____
COLD	chronic obstructive lung disease	_____
COPD	chronic obstructive pulmonary disease	_____
CP	cerebral palsy	_____
CPD	cephalopelvic disproportion	_____
CRF	chronic renal failure	_____
CT	carpal tunnel	_____
	coronary thrombosis	_____
CVA	cerebrovascular accident	_____
CVD	cardiovascular disease	_____
DOA	dead on arrival	_____
DRG	Diagnostic Related Groups	_____
DTs	delirium tremens	_____
Dx	diagnosis	_____

(Continued)

DIAGNOSES

ESRD	end-stage renal failure	
FB	foreign body	
FOD	free of disease	
FTND	full-term normal delivery	
FTT	failure to thrive	
FUO	fever of unknown origin	
Fx	fracture	
FxBB	fracture both bones	
GNID	gram-negative intracellular diplococci	
Grav I/ab I	one pregnancy/one abortion	
HA	headache	
	hearing aid	
	hemolytic anemia	
HAA	hepatitis-associated antigen	
HC	Huntington's chorea	
HCVD	hypertensive cardiovascular disease	
HD	Hodgkin's disease	
HDN	hemolytic disease of newborn	
HF	heart failure	
HH	hiatal hernia	
HLV	herpes-like virus	
HSV	herpes simplex virus	
HTLV-III/LAV	Human T-cell lymphotropic virus III/	
	Lymphadenopathy associated virus	
IHD	ischemic heart disease	
IM	infectious mononucleosis	
JOB	juvenile-onset diabetes	
LE	lupus erythematosus	
LGB	Landry-Guillan-Barré syndrome	
MBD	minimal brain dysfunction	
MD	manic depressive	
	muscular dystrophy	
	myocardial disease	
met, metas	metastases	
MVP	mitral valve prolapse	
MOD	maturity onset diabetes	
Mono	mononucleosis	
MS	mitral stenosis	
	multiple sclerosis	
OA	osteoarthritis	
OAG	open-angle glaucoma	

(Continued)

351

DIAGNOSES

OM	otitis media	_____
PAR	perennial allergic rhinitis	_____
para	paraplegic	_____
para (I, II)	one live birth (two . . .)	_____
PCD	polycystic disease	_____
PD	Parkinson's disease	_____
	pulmonary disease	_____
PKU	phenylketonuria	_____
PND	paroxysmal nocturnal dyspnea	_____
preg	pregnant	_____
PVC	premature ventricular contraction	_____
PE	pulmonary edema	_____
S–C disease	sickle cell hemoglobin-c disease	_____
schiz	schizophrenia	_____
SIDS	sudden infant death syndrome	_____
TB	tuberculosis, tuberculin bacillus	_____
Thal	thalassemia	_____
TIA	transischemic attack	_____
TSD	Tay-Sachs disease	_____
URI	upper respiratory disease	_____
UTI	urinary tract infection	_____

PROCEDURES

AB	abortion	_____
A + P	auscultation and percussion	_____
ABO	blood typing groups	_____
ACTH	adrenocortiotropic hormone (test)	_____
AFB	acid-fast bacillus	_____
ANA	antinuclear antibodies	_____
BE, BaE	barium enema	_____
BCG	immunization, B-scan sonogram	_____
BP	blood pressure	_____
BUN	blood urea nitrogen	_____
Bx, Bl	biopsy	_____
CAB	coronary artery bypass	_____
CAD	computer-aided design	_____
CBC	complete blood count	_____
CAPD	chronic ambulatory peritoneal dialysis	_____
Ch, Chol	cholesterol	_____
CPK	creatine phosphokinase	_____
CPR	cardiopulmonary resuscitation	_____
C + S	culture and sensitivity	_____

(Continued)

PROCEDURES

C section	Cesarean section	
CT	computed tomography	
CXR	chest x-ray	
Cysto	cystoscopy	
CPAP	continuous positive airway pressure ventilation	
CSF	cerebrospinal fluid	
D & C	dilation and curettage	
Del	delivery	
DHT	dihydrotestosterone	
DNA	deoxyribonucleic acid	
DPT	diphtheria pertussis	
ECG, EKG	electrocardiogram	
ECHO	echocardiogram	
ECT	electroconvulsive therapy	
EEG	electroencephalogram	
EMIT	enzyme immunoassay for drug screening	
EMG	electromyogram	
ERG	electroretinogram	
ex	excise	
exam	examination	
FBS	fasting blood sugar	
FME	full-mouth extraction	
FSH	follicle-stimulating hormone	
GA	gastric analysis	
GT, GTT	glucose tolerance test	
GxT	graded exercise test	
HAA	hepatitis Australian antigen	
HAI	hemagglutination inhibition– rubella test	
Hb, Hgb	hemoglobin	
Hct	hematocrit	
HDL	high-density lipoproteins	
H + P	history and physical	
HGH	human growth hormone	
HSG	hysterosalpingogram	
Hx	history	
IABP	intra-aortic balloon pump	
ICSH	interstitial cell stimulating hormone	
ICAT	indirect Coomb's test	
I + D	incision and drainage	
IPPB	intermittent positive-pressure breathing	

(Continued)

PROCEDURES

IVP	intravenous pyelogram	_____
KUB	kidney ureter bladder (x-ray)	_____
lab	laboratory	_____
LASER	light amplification by stimulated emission of radiation	_____
LDH	lactose dehydrogenase	_____
LP	lumbar puncture	_____
LH	luteinizing hormone	_____
LOS	length of stay	_____
MASER	microwave amplification by stimulated emission of radiation	_____
MMRV	measles, mumps, rubella vaccine	_____
OC	office call	_____
O + P	ova and parasites test	_____
OPG	oculoplethysmography	_____
P + A	percussion and auscultation	_____
Pap	Papanicolaou test	_____
PBI	protein-bound iodine	_____
PCV	packed cell volume	_____
PE	physical exam	_____
pH	hydrogen ion concentration, acid/base	_____
Pt, protime	prothrombin time	_____
PTT	partial thromboplastin time	_____
2hr pc	2-hour postcibal blood glucose	_____
2 hr pg	2-hour postglucose blood glucose	_____
2hr pp	2-hour postprandial blood glucose	_____
P + V	pyloroplasty and vagotomy	_____
RIA	radioimmunoassay	_____
RPR	syphills test (also: DRT, VDRL, STS)	_____
RATx	radiation therapy	_____
Rx	take, prescribe	_____
RPG	retrograde pyelogram	_____
SGOT	serum glutamic oxaloacetic transaminase	_____
SGPT	serum glutamic pyruvic transaminase	
SOP	standard operating procedure	_____
Sp gr	specific gravity (urine)	_____
T3, T4	thyroid test	_____
T	temperature	_____
TSH	thyroid-stimulating hormone	_____

(Continued)

PROCEDURES

TAA	total abdominal hysterectomy	_____
TENS	transcutaneous electrical nerve stimulation	_____
TUR	transurethral resection	_____
Tx	treatment	_____
XM	cross-match for blood	_____
XR	x-ray	_____
VCG	vectorcardiogram	_____
VDRL	syphilis test	_____
YAG	yttrium aluminum garnet (laser)	_____
V, Y, W, Z, -plasty	various types of procedures used to repair lacerations	_____

HEALTH PROFESSIONS

AAMA	American Association of Medical Assistants	_____
AMA	American Medical Association	_____
AOA	American Osteopathic Association	_____
ASCP	American Society of Clinical Pathology	_____
CMA	Certified Medical Assistant	_____
CPHA	Commission on Professional and Hospital Activities	_____
DDS	Doctor of Dental Surgery	_____
DC	Doctor of Chiropractic	_____
DO	Doctor of Osteopathy	_____
DPM	Doctor of Podiatric Medicine	_____
EENT	Eye, Ear, Nose, and Throat specialist	_____
EMT	Emergency Medical Technician	_____
ENT	Ear, Nose, and Throat specialist	_____
FACP	Fellow of the American College of Physicians	_____
FACS	Fellow of the American College of Surgeons	_____
GYN	gynecology	_____
LPN	Licensed Practical Nurse	_____
LVN	Licensed Vocational Nurse	_____
MD	medical doctor	_____
MT	medical technologist	_____
NP	nurse practitioner	_____
ORTH	orthopedist	_____
OB	obstetrician	_____

(Continued)

HEALTH PROFESSIONS

OT	occupational therapist	_____
PA	physician's assistant	_____
PC	professional corporation	_____
PT	physical therapy	_____
RRA	Registered Records Administrator	_____
RRT	Registered Radiography Technician	_____
RT	respiratory therapist	_____

CHARTING ABBREVIATIONS

aa	of each	_____
ac	before meals	_____
ad	right ear (auricle dexter)	_____
aj	ankle jerk	_____
adm	admission	_____
ant	anterior	_____
am	mornings	_____
approx	approximately	_____
AP	anteroposterior	_____
AV	atrioventricular	_____
ax	axillary	_____
bid	twice a day (bis in die)	_____
bin	twice a night (bis in noctus)	_____
BMR	basal metabolism rate	_____
BM	bowel movement	_____
BP	blood pressure	_____
$\bar{c}$, /w	with	_____
C1, C2, C3, . . .	cervical vertebra first, second, third, . . .	_____
C	centigrade	_____
cap(s)	capsules	_____
CC	chief complaint	_____
CCU	cardiac care unit	_____
c/o	complains of	_____
cont	continue	_____
D	diopter (ocular measure)	_____
dc	discontinue	_____
DC	discharge from hospital	_____
Dr	doctor	_____
Dx	diagnosis	_____
DNA	does not apply	_____

(Continued)

CHARTING ABBREVIATIONS

DNS	did not show	_____
EOM	extraocular movements	_____
Ex	examination	_____
F	Fahrenheit	_____
fhs	fetal heart sounds	_____
fht	fetal heart tones	_____
GB	gall bladder	_____
GI	gastrointestinal	_____
GU	genitourinary	_____
hpf	high-power field	_____
hs	hour of sleep, bedtime (hora somni)	_____
hypo	hypodermically	_____
ICU	intensive care unit	_____
IM	intramuscular	_____
I + O	intake and output	_____
iss	one and one half	_____
IV	intravenous	_____
L	left	_____
L1, L2, L3, . . .	lumbar vertebrae first, second, third, . . .	_____
L + A	light and accommodation	_____
L + W	living and well	_____
lmp	last menstrual period	_____
lpf	low-power field (10 ×)	_____
LUQ	left upper quadrant of abdomen	_____
MTD	right eardrum (membrana tympani dexter)	_____
MTS	left eardrum (membrana tympani sinister)	_____
NPO	nothing by mouth	_____
neg	negative	_____
OD	right eye (oculus dexter)	_____
OLA	occipital lay anterior (fetal presentation)	_____
OP	outpatient	_____
OS	left eye (oculus sinister)	_____
OU	both eyes (oculus uterque)	_____
P	pulse	_____
PA	posteroanterior	_____
pc	after meals (post cibum)	_____
PDR	Physician's Desk Reference	_____

357

(Continued)

CHARTING ABBREVIATIONS

Pl	present illness	
po	by mouth, postoperative	
pm	afternoon or evening	
prn	as needed or desired (pro re nata)	
q	every (quaque)	
qh	every hour	
q2h	every two hours	
qid	four times a day (quarter in die)	
qm	every morning	
qn	every night	
R	right, respiration	
RBC	red blood cell, erythrocyte count	
Rh	blood factor, Rh$^+$ or Rh$^-$	
RLQ	right lower quadrant (abdomen)	
RO, R/O	rule out	
RUQ	right upper quadrant (abdomen)	
$\bar{s}$, w/o	without (sans)	
sc, subcu	subcutaneously (into fat layer)	
sed rate	sedimentation rate (blood)	
SOB	short of breath	
ss	half	
staph	staphylococcus	
stat	immediately (statum)	
strep	streptococcus	
T1, T2, T3, . . .	thoracic vertebrae first, second, third, . . .	
T	temperature	
tab(s)	tablets	
tid	three times a day	
tinct	tincture	
ULQ	upper left quadrant (abdomen)	
ung	ointment (unguentum)	
URQ	upper right quadrant (abdomen)	
WBC	white blood cell, leukocyte count	
WM, BM	white male, black male	

(Continued)

358

CHARTING ABBREVIATIONS

WF, BF	white female, black female	_____
x	times, power	_____
y/o, yrs	years old	_____
+	positive	_____
−	negative	_____
♀	female	_____
♂	male	_____
+/−	positive or negative	_____
*	birth	_____
†	death	_____
p̄	after	_____
ā	before	_____
↑	increase	_____
↓	decrease	_____
>	greater than	_____
<	less than	_____

359

INDEX OF TERMS

Note: Indexing is by frame number.

antinarcotic, 1176
antipyretic, 1175
antirheumatic, 1178
antiseptic, 1180
antitoxic, 1179
antitoxin, 1175
anuresis, 1144
anuria, 1144
aortic, 1200
apepsia, 561
apex, 1278
aphasia, 784
aphonia, 787
aplasia, 826
apnea, 543, 1144
aponeurosis, 1272
appendicitis, 1277
arachnoid, 325
areflexia, 1141
arteriectasia, 765
arteriofibrosis, 569
arteriomalacia, 569
arteriorrhexis, 771
arteriosclerosis, 268, 568,
  763
arteriospasm, 570
arteriostasis, 954, 1379
arthritis, 348
arthroplasty, 344
arthroscope, 342
arthroscopy, 343
arthrotomy, 349
asepsis, 1144, 1170
aseptic, 1171
atrium, 1266
autodermic, 1018
autodiagnosis, 1018
autohemotherapy, 1021
autoimmunity, 1016
autolysis, 1019
autonephrectomy, 1022
autonomic, 1019
autophagia, 1020
autophilia, 1118
autophobia, 1020
autoplasty, 1021
autopsy, 1113
autopsychosis, 1021

bicellular, 1220
bicuspid, 1216

bifocal, 1216
bifurcate, 1223
bifurcation, 1216, 1224
bilateral, 1218
binuclear, 1221
biochemistry, 924
biogenesis, 925
biologist, 925
biology, 925
biopsy, 932
bipara, 1222
blastoderm, 988
blepharedema, 1447
blepharitis, 1448
blepharoplasty, 1449
blepharoptosis, 1446
blepharorrhaphy, 668
blepharospasm, 1449
blepharotomy, 1448
botulism, 930
bradycardia, 525
bradykinesia, 796, 803
bradypepsia, 561
bradyphagia, 526
bradyphasia, 784
bradypnea, 538, 545
bronchiectasis, 483
bronchitis, 1308
broncholith, 1309
bronchopneumonia, 483
bronchorrhagia, 1309
bronchorrhaphy, 1310
bronchoscope, 1308
bronchoscopy, 1309
bronchospasm, 1310
bronchostomy, 1310
bursa, 351, 1255
bursectomy, 351
bursitis, 351

"c" rule, 460
calcaneal, 1388
calcaneodynia, 1388
calcaneum, 1385
calculus, 508
carcinogenesis, 551
carcinoma, 261–265
cardialgia, 189
cardiocentesis, 428
cardiologist, 180
cardiology, 180

cardiomegaly, 165
cardiometer, 401
cardiorrhexis, 770
carpal, 1166, 1393
carpectomy, 1393
carpoptosis, 1393
carpus, 1390
cartilage, 353
catarrh, 505
cauda, 921
caudal, 905
caudate, 921
caudation, 921
centesis, 426
cephalad, 920
cephalalgia, 281
cephalic, 288, 903
cephalodynia, 283
cephalodynic, 285
cephalometer, 401, 920
cephalotripsy, 920
cerebral, 317
cerebritis, 319
cerebroma, 320, 1071
cerebropathy, 341
cerebrospinal, 322
cerebrotomy, 321
cerebrum, 314
cervical, 1283
cervicectomy, 1283
cervicitis, 1283
cerviobrachial, 1285
cervicofacial, 1285
cervicovesical, 1285
cervix, 1281
cheilitis, 721
cheiloplasty, 721
cheilosis, 723
cheilostomatoplasty, 724
cheilotomy, 723
chicken pox, 889
chiromegaly,
chiroplasty, 1330
chiropractic, 1331
chiropractor, 1331
chirospasm, 1328
chloremia, 138
chlorocyte, 136
chloropia, 1444
cholecyst, 517
cholecystectomy, 521
cholecystitis, 518

cholecystotomy, 521
cholelith, 513
cholelithotomy, 521
cholestasis, 1377
cholesterol, 268
chondralgia, 354
chondrectomy, 356
chondrocostal, 357, 360
chondrodynia, 354
chondrodysplasia, 828
chromoblast, 934
chromocyte, 934
chromogenesis, 935
chromolysis, 935
chromometer, 935
chromophilic, 936–939
ciliary body, 1476
circumduction, 1096
circumocular, 1091
circumoral, 1092
circumscribed, 1093
clot, 587
coccus, 467
colic, 734
colocentesis, 734
coloclysis, 736
colopexy, 735
coloptosis, 736
colostomy, 735
colpectomy, 617
colpitis, 615
colpodynia, 616
colpopathy, 616
colpopexy, 618
colpoplasty, 618
colpoptosis, 650
colporrhaphy, 668
colposcope, 619
colpospasm, 617
colpotomy, 619
conductivity, 1517
condyle, 1420
condylectomy, 1421
condyloid, 1421
congenital, 1232
conjunctiva, 1255
consanguinity, 1239
contraceptive, 1186
contraction, 1512
contraindicated, 1187
contraindication, 1186
contralateral, 1186

contrary, 1182
contravolitional, 1186
corectasia, 1469
corectopia, 1469
corelysis, 1469
coreometer, 1470
coreometry, 1470
coreoplasty, 1470
cornea, 1450
corneitis, 1451
corneoiritis, 1451, 1458
corneosclera, 1451
cortical, 1277
costal, 362
costectomy, 358
cranial, 311
craniectomy, 308
craniocerebral, 313
craniomalacia, 307
craniometer, 310
cranioplasty, 306
craniotomy, 309
crypt, 594
cryptectomy, 594
cryptitis, 594
cryptogram, 593
cryptopyic, 595
cryptorchidism, 589,
   591, 1508
cryptorrhea, 596
cryptotoxic, 593
cyanemia, 138
cyanoderma, 134, 135
cyanopia, 814, 1444
cyanosis, 58, 126, 1114
cyanotic, 58, 60, 114
cycloplegia, 1477
cyst, 861
cystectomy, 434
cystocele, 435
cystoplasty, 444
cystorrhagia, 674, 774
cystorrhaphy, 667, 774
cystorrhea, 774
cystorrhexis, 769, 774
cystotomy, 433
cyte, 136
cytology, 147
cytolysis, 571
cytometer, 401, 1493
cytometry, 1493
cytophagocytosis, 1491

cytophagy, 1492
cytoscopy, 1494
cytostasis, 1494

dacryoadenalgia, 1488
dacryocystitis, 1488
dacryocystocele, 1489
dacryocystoptosis, 1490
dacryocystotome, 1490
dacryolith, 1489
dacryoma, 1488
dacryorrhea, 1486, 1490
dacryopyorrhea, 1489
dactylitis, 869
dactylogram, 869
dactylomegaly, 868
dactylospasm, 869
Darwinism, 1510
decalcification, 1054
deciduous, 1048
decoction, 1049
dehydration, 1050
delirium, 1266
dentalgia, 373
dentifrice, 375
dentoid, 374
dermatitis, 123
dermatologist, 111
dermatome, 131
dermatomycosis, 701
dermatosis, 125
dermic, 237
dermopathy, 133
dextrad, 1323
dextral, 1324
dextrocardia, 1324
dextrogastria, 1324
dextromanual, 1325
dextropedal, 1325
diagnosis, 848
dialysis, 849, 852
diaphragm, 1315
diarrhea, 850, 1099
diascope, 857
diathermal, 1099
diathermic, 1099
diathermy, 851, 855
digestible, 1522
digit, 869
diplobacterium, 813
diploblastic,

diplocardiac, 804
diplococcus, 465, 813
diplogenesis, 804
diplopia, 805, 1445
dipsomania, 894
dipsomaniac, 895
dipsosis, 896
dipsotherapy, 896
disassociate, 1245
disease, 1242
disinfect, 1244
disinfectant, 1244
dissect, 1243
dissection, 1243
dissociate, 1245
dorsal, 901
dorsocephalad, 911
dorsodynia, 911
dromomania, 881
duodenal, 60, 215
duodenitis, 211
duodenocholecystostomy, 761
duodenotomy, 207
duodenum, 59, 200, 759
dura mater, 325
dysentery, 947, 948
dysesthesia, 777, 942
dyskinesia, 942
dysmenorrhea, 554, 951
dyspepsia, 558, 559, 941
dyspeptic, 941
dysphagia, 555
dysphasia, 785
dysphonia, 785
dysphoria, 942, 1372
dysplasia, 825
dyspnea, 556, 941
dystocia, 943
dystrophy, 556

ectocytic, 999
ectoderm, 988
ectogenous, 998
ectopic, 1003
ectoplasm, 1000
electrocardiogram, 185–187
electrocardiograph, 186
elephantiasis, 516
embryonic, 563, 1343

emesis, 242, 945
encephalitis, 227, 292
encephalocele, 295
encephaloma, 293
encephalomalacia, 228, 301
encephalomeningitis, 229
encephalomyelopathy, 230
encephalorrhagia, 673
encephalotomy, 304
endocardiac, 1002
endocardial, 1002
endochondral, 1001
endocolitis, 1002
endocranial, 1001
endocrinologist, 1542
endocystic, 999
endoderm, 988
endoenteritis, 1002
endogenous, 998
endometritis, 641
endometrium, 641, 1004
endoplasm, 1000
enterectasia, 732
enterocele, 731
enterocentesis, 733
enterocholecystostomy, 760
enterocyclis, 731
enteroplegia, 732
enteroptosis, 733
enterorrhagia, 730
enterorrhexis, 769
enteroscope, 737
enterostasis, 1378
epicondyle, 1421
epicranial, 1149
epicystitis, 1147
epidermal, 1149
epigastric, 1145
epigastrorrhaphy, 1148
epinephrectomy, 48
epinephritis, 1147
episplenitis, 1146
episternal, 1149
erythremia, 138
erythroblast, 137
erythrocyte, 136, 157
erythrocytopenia, 157
erythroderma, 135
erythropia, 1444
esophagoduodenostomy, 759
esophagogastroscopy, 761

esophagogastrostomy, 760
esophagus, 759
esophoria, 1369
esthesia, 775
esthesiometer, 776
esthesioscopy, 776
euesthesia, 942
eugenics, 946
eukinesia, 942
eupepsia, 941
eupeptic, 941
euphoria, 942, 1372
eupnea, 941
euthanasia, 945, 946
eutocia, 943
excretion, 1060–1062
exeresis, 1058
exhale, 1059
exophoria, 1369
expiration, 1195
extra-articular, 1152
extracerebral, 1153
extracystic, 1152
extradural, 1152
extragenital, 1153
extrahepatic, 1153
extranuclear, 1150
extrauterine, 1151

fallopian tubes, 610, 630
febrile, 1251
fetal alcohol syndrome, 884
focus, 1258
fornix, 1278
fossa, 1255
fungistasis, 1376
fungus, 697

"g" rule, 620
gallbladder, 244, 515, 517, 518
gallstone, 515
ganglion, 1270, 1423
gangrene, 1110, 1111
gastralgia, 190
gastrectasia, 728
gastrectomy, 193
gastric, 728
gastritis, 197, 728

gastroduodenostomy, 201, 218
gastroenteric, 730
gastroenterocolostomy, 760
gastroenteroptosis, 729
gastromalacia, 570
gastromegaly, 170, 198
gastrorrhagia, 673, 728
gastrospasm, 570
genesis, 547
geriatrician, 1549
gingival, 725
gingivalgia, 726
gingivectomy, 727
gingivitis, 726
gingivoglossitis, 727
glaucoma, 1236
glossal, 717
glossalgia, 717
glossectomy, 716
glossitis, 716
glossoplegia, 720
glossoplegic, 720
glossoptosis, 719
glossoscopy, 719
glucose, 980
glycemia, 983
glycogen, 980
glycogenesis, 985
glycolipid, 987
glycolysis, 986
glycorrhea, 986
gnathalgia, 947
gnathitis, 946
gnathodynia, 947
gnathoplasty, 948
gnoses, 843
gnosia, 843
gumma, 1269
gynecoid, 653
gynecologic, 652
gynecological, 652
gynecologist, 652
gynecology, 651
gynecopathy, 653
gynecophobia, 653

heartburn, 151
hemangiitis, 572
hemarthrosis, 572

hematologist, 574
hematology, 574
hematolysis, 573
hematophilia, 1117
hematophobia, 573
hemiatrophy, 1231
hemicardia, 1229
hemidystrophy, 1231
hemigastrectomy, 1229
hemihypertrophy, 1231
hemiparalysis, 1229
hemiplegia, 1229
hemodialysis, 849
hemoglobin, 156
hemolysis, 571, 573
hemorrhage, 673
hemostasis, 953, 1379
hepatalgia, 754
hepatectomy, 749
hepatic, 747
hepatocele, 754
hepatodynia, 754
hepatolith, 754
hepatomegaly, 747
hepatopathy, 748
hepatorrhaphy, 753, 773
hepatorrhea, 773
hepatorrhexis, 773
hepatoscopy, 748
hepatotomy, 749
heterogeneous, 1129
heterogenesis, 1130
heterolyses, 1130
heteropia, 1127
heterosexual, 1128
hidroadenitis, 976
hidrocystoma, 975
hidrorrhea, 977
hidrosis, 977
histoblast, 1343
histocyte, 1343
histogenous, 1341
histoid, 1343
histologist, 1342
histology, 1342
histolysis, 1340
histoma, 1342
homogeneous, 1129
homogenesis, 1130
homogenized, 1121
homoglandular, 1121
homolateral, 1123

homolysis, 1130
homosexual, 1124
homothermal, 1122
humeral, 1418
humeroradical, 1418
humeroscapular, 1418
humeroulnar, 1418
humerus, 1417
hydrocephalic, 449
hydrocephalus, 446, 859
hydrocephaly, 297
hydrocyst, 445
hydrophilia, 1117
hydrophobia, 450, 1117
hydrophthalmos, 1236
hydrotherapy, 455
hyoid, 1248
hyperalgesia, 780
hyperemesis, 242
hyperemesis gravidarum, 243
hyperemia, 1528
hyperesthesia, 778
hyperglycemia, 984
hyperhidrosis, 977
hyperopia, 814, 1445
hyperphasia, 785
hyperphoria, 1371
hyperplasia, 826
hyperthyroidism, 241, 1509
hypertrophy, 236, 245
hypodermic, 237–240
hypoesthesia, 777
hypoglossal, 718
hypoglycemia, 984
hypophonia, 785
hypophoria, 1371
hypopituitarism, 1511
hypoplasia, 827
hypotrophy, 234
hysterectomy, 631
hysteria, 837
hysterocele, 640, 643
hysteropathy, 633, 640
hysteropexy, 633, 643
hysteroptosis, 645
hysterorrhexis, 767
hysterosalpingo-
  oophorectomy, 634
hysterospasm, 632
hysterotomy, 632

ileocecal, 1199
ileum, 1266
immunity, 1016, 1017
incise, 1203
incision, 1203
incompatible, 1197
incompetency, 1198
incompetent, 1201
inflatable, 1523
infracostal, 1162
inframammary, 1156
infrapatellar, 1157
infrapubic, 1163
infrasternal, 1161
inject, 1205
injection, 1205
insane, 1207
insanitary, 1207
insomnia, 1207
inspiration, 1195
interchondral, 364
intercostal, 363
interdental, 368
intra-abdominal, 1261
intra-arterial, 1264
intracellular, 1262
intracranial, 1264
intracystic, 1264
intradermal, 1265
intraduodenal, 1265
intralumbar, 1263
intraspinal, 1263
intrathoracic, 1265
intravenous, 1076, 1263
iridalgia, 1461
iridectomy, 1461
iridocele, 1461
iridomalacia, 1462
iridoparalysis, 1463
iridoplegia, 1463
iridoptosis, 1462
iridorrhexis, 1462
irides, 1459
iris, 1457
iritis, 1458
irritability, 1518
ischemia, 1527
ischial, 1400
ischiocele, 1400
ischioneuralgia, 1399
ischiopubic, 1399
ischiorectal, 1399

ischium, 1396
isocellular, 1074
isodactylism, 1078, 1509
isometric, 1073
isothermal, 1078
isothermic, 1078
isotonic, 1075

jejunoileostomy, 761

keratectasia, 1474
keratocele, 1474
keratoplasty, 1474
keratorrhexis, 1475
keratoscleritis, 1475
keratotomy, 1475
kinesia, 878
kinesialgia, 797
kinesiology, 800
Korsakoff's syndrome, 883

lacrimal, 1481
lacrimation, 1486
laparectomy, 966
laparocolostomy, 969
laparogastrotomy, 969
laparohepatotomy, 969
laparohysterosalpingo-
  oophorectomy, 970
laparorrhaphy, 968
laparoscopy, 967
laparotomy, 968
laryngalgia, 1298
laryngitis, 1297
laryngocele, 1302
laryngopathy, 1303
laryngoscope, 1303
laryngospasm, 1303
laryngostomy, 1299
laryngotomy, 1300
larynx, 1296
lateral, 896
leukemia, 154, 1527
leukoblast, 137
leukocyte, 136, 148
leukocytopenia, 151
leukoderma, 135, 143
lipoid, 266
lipolysis, 571
lipoma, 259
lithiasis, 515, 821
lithogenesis, 509

lithology, 510
lithometer, 511
lithotomy, 511
lithotripsy, 821
locus, 1258
lumbar, 1263
lymphostasis, 954

macroblast, 865
macrocephalus, 865
macrocheilia, 866
macrococcus, 865
macrocyte, 864
macrodactylia, 867
macroglossia, 866
macrophage, 1506
macrorhinia, 866
macroscopic, 864
macrotia, 866
macules, 889
malacotomy, 305
malaise, 1210
malaria, 1212
malarial, 1213
malariology, 1213
malariotherapy, 1213
malformation, 1210
malignant, 261
malnutrition, 1211
malodorous, 1209
malposition, 1211
mania, 174
maxilla, 1279
medical dictionary, 94
megalocardia, 164
megalogastria, 168, 198
megalomania, 175
melanin, 692
melanoblast, 137
melanocarcinoma, 694
melanocyte, 136, 692
melanoderma, 135, 693
melanoma, 691, 1347
melanosis, 691
menarche, 951
Mendelism, 1510
meninges, 325
meningitis, 325
meningocele, 327
meningococci, 330
meningomalacia, 328
menopause, 950

menorrhagia, 950
menorrhea, 951
menostasis, 952
menses, 949
mesocardia, 1006
mesocephalic, 1006
mesocolic, 1006
mesoderm, 989
mesoneuritis, 1006
metacarpals, 1166
metastasis, 1168
metatarsis, 1167
metritis, 638
metrocele, 640
metroparalysis, 638
metropathy, 640
metrorrhagia, 639
metrorrhea, 639
metrorrhexis, 772
microcardia, 861
microcephalus, 859
microcyst, 861
microcyte, 861
microphage, 1506
microscope, 45, 857
microsurgery, 862
monilia, 516
moniliasis, 516
monocyte, 1025
monoma, 1025
monomania, 1025
monomyoplegia, 1026
mononeural, 1026
mononuclear, 1024
mononucleosis, 1026
mucoid, 269
mucosa, 277
mucous, 58, 273, 1519
mucus, 58, 273
multicapsular, 1029
multicellular, 1030, 1220
multiglandular, 1030
multinuclear, 1030
multipara, 1031, 1222
multiparous, 1031, 1032
myasthenia, 791
mycelium, 698
mycoid, 700
mycology, 700
mycosis, 699
myelitis, 822
myeloblast, 823

myelocele, 824
myelocytic, 824
myelodysplasia, 824
myoblast, 563
myobradia, 791
myocarditis, 789
myocardium, 791
myofibroma, 566, 792
myofibrosis, 792
myofibrositis, 792
myogram, 790
myograph, 790
myography, 790
myoid, 793
myolipoma, 793
myolysis, 567
myopathy, 793
myopia, 1445
myosclerosis, 565
myospasm, 564

narcolepsy, 1069
narcosis, 1068
narcotic, 1064
naris, 1273
nasal, 1289
nasitis, 1289
nasoantritis, 1287
nasofrontal, 1290
nasolacrimal, 1290, 1484
nasomental, 1288
nasopharyngeal, 1291
nasopharyngitis, 1290
nasoscope, 1289
navel, 913–919
necrectomy, 1112
necrocytosis, 1107
necroparasite, 1108
necrophilia, 1116
necrophobia, 1112, 1116
necropsy, 1113
necrosis, 1109, 1114
necrotic, 1114
necrotomy, 1112
nematode worm, 516
neocyte, 1349
neogenesis, 1344
neonatal, 1345
neopathy, 1349
neophobia, 1349
neoplasm, 1345

nephritis, 656
nephrolith, 657
nephrolysis, 656
nephromalacia, 657
nephromegaly, 657
nephropexy, 656
nephroptosis, 654
nephrorrhaphy, 667
nervous, 58, 1520
neuralgia, 815
neurasthenia, 837
neuritis, 818
neuroarthropathy, 816
neuroblast, 563
neurofibroma, 566
neurologist, 817
neurology, 817
neurolysis, 567, 818
neuromyelitis, 829
neuroplasty, 818
neurorrhaphy, 668
neurosclerosis, 565
neurospasm, 564
neurotripsy, 819
noctambulism, 1352
noctiluca, 1350
noctiphilia, 1360
noctiphobia, 1360
nocturia, 1362
nullipara, 1036
nyctalbuminuria, 1356
nyctalgia, 1355
nyctalopia, 1357
nyctophilia, 1360
nyctophobia, 1360
nycturia, 1361

obstetrics, 1548
omphalectomy, 917
omphalic, 917
omphalitis, 914
omphalocele, 917
omphalorrhagia, 918
omphalorrhea, 918
omphalorrhexis, 918
oncology, 1543
onychocryptosis, 1500
onychoid, 1497
onychoma, 1497
onychomalacia, 1498
onychomycosis, 1498

onychophagia, 1498, 1507
onychosis, 1497
ooblast, 597
oogenesis, 598
oophorectomy, 603
oophoritis, 604
oophoro, 600
oophoroma, 604
oophoropexy, 605
ophthalmalgia, 1438
ophthalmic, 1437
ophthalmitis, 1437
ophthalmocele, 1440
ophthalmodynia, 1438
ophthalmologist, 1442
ophthalmology, 1442
ophthalmometer, 1440
ophthalmopathy, 1441
ophthalmoplasty, 1441
ophthalmoplegia, 1441
ophthalmoscope, 1443
ophthalmoscopy, 1443
orchidalgia, 588
orchidectomy, 588
orchidocele, 590
orchidopexy, 590, 609
orchidoplasty, 589
orchidotomy, 590
orthopedics, 1550
osteitis, 332
osteoarthropathy, 339, 340
osteochondritis, 352
osteochondrodysplasia, 828
osteoma, 338
osteomalacia, 333
osteopathy, 331
otalgia, 495
otitis media, 494
otodynia, 495
otorhinolaryngologist, 1547
otorrhea, 491
ovary, 601
ovum, 597, 630

palatoschisis, 1382
pancreatectomy, 752
pancreatic, 750
pancreatolith, 751
pancreatolysis, 750

pancreatopathy, 751
pancreatotomy, 752
para-appendicitis, 1011
paracentesis, 424
paracentral, 1011
paracolpitis, 1012
paracystitis, 1012
parahepatitis, 781, 1013
paralgesia, 780
paralgia, 780
paralysis, 782
paranephritis, 781, 1013
paraosteoarthropathy, 783
paraphasia, 784
paraplegia, 782
parasalpingitis, 783
paresis, 1071
pediatrics, 1550
pelvimeter, 397
pelvimetry, 394
pelvis, 393, 1272
percussion, 1105
perforate, 1101
perforation, 1100
periadenitis, 1089
periarticular, 1086
pericardiectomy, 1089
perichondral, 1088
pericolic, 1087
pericolpitis, 1089
peridental, 1088
perihepatitis, 1089
peritonsillar, 1086
phagocyte, 1505
phagocytosis, 1505
phalangectomy, 1412
phalanges, 1410
phalangitis, 1412
phalanx, 1412
pharyngitis, 1294
pharyngocele, 1294
pharyngolith, 1292
pharyngomycosis, 701, 1293
pharyngopathy, 1295
pharyngoplasty, 1295
pharyngoscope, 1295
pharyngotomy, 1294
pharynx, 1286
phlebectasia, 765
phlebectomy, 764
phlebopexy, 764
phleboplasty, 766

phleborrhexis, 771
phlebosclerosis, 763
phlebostasis, 953, 1379
phlebotomy, 766
phobia, 451, 573
phonic, 787
phonocardiography, 788
phonology, 788
phonometer, 787
phonomyogram, 788
phonomyography, 788
phorology, 1374
phorometer, 1370
phrenectomy, 1316
phrenoplegia, 1315
pia mater, 325
pleura, 1256
pleural, 1311
pleuralgia, 1312
pleurectomy, 1313
pleurisy, 1314
pleuritis, 1311
pleurocentesis, 1312
pleurodynia, 1312
pleurolith, 1313
pleurovisceral, 1313
plural words, 1254
pneopneic, 536
pneumococcus, 463
pneumoderma, 705
pneumohemothorax, 709
pneumometer, 708
pneumonectomy, 681
pneumonia, 463, 683
pneumonitis, 685
pneumonocentesis, 684
pneumonomelanosis, 687
pneumonomycosis, 696, 699
pneumonopathy, 682
pneumonopexy, 686
pneumonorrhagia, 682
pneumonotomy, 681
pneumopyothorax, 709
pneumoserothorax, 719
pneumotherapy, 707
pneumothoracic, 706
pneumothorax, 705
podalgia, 1326
podiatric, 1329
podiatrist, 1327, 1329
polyarthritis, 873
polycystic, 874

polydactylism, 870
polydipsia, 890
polyneuralgia, 873
polyneuropathy, 872
polyotia, 873
polyphagia, 874
polyphobia, 874
polyuria, 871
postcibal, 1247
posterior, 906
posteroexternal, 910
posterointernal, 910
posterolateral, 910
postesophageal, 1247
postfebrile, 1251
postmortem, 1113, 1260
postnatal, 1250
postoperative, 1252
postparalytic, 1252
postpartum, 1252
postuterine, 1252
preanesthetic, 1248
precancerous, 1253
prefrontal, 1253
prehyoid, 1248
prenatal, 1250
preoperative, 1253
preparalytic, 1253
presbyopia, 1445
primipara, 1036
procephalic, 846
proctoclysis, 744
proctologist, 743
proctopexy, 746
protoplegia, 744
proctorrhaphy, 746
proctoscope, 745
proctoscopy, 745
prodromal, 888, 889
prodrome, 886
prognosis, 844
prognostic, 846
prolapse, 644
protoplasm, 1000
protozoon, 1270
pseudocyesis, 958
pseudocyst, 960
pseudoedema, 960
pseudoesthesia, 960
pseudohypertrophy, 961
pseudomania, 959
pseudoparalysis, 959

pseudoscience, 958
pseudosyphilis, 961
pseudotuberculosis, 961
psychasthenia, 837
psychiatrist, 832, 1332, 1515
psychiatry, 832
psychoanalysis, 831
psychogenesis, 834
psychologist, 833
psychology, 833
psychoneurosis, 835
psychopath, 838
psychopathic, 838
psychopathy, 838
psychopharmacology, 841
psychosis, 834
psychosomatic, 831
psychosurgery, 831
psychotherapy, 832
ptosis, 646
pubic, 391
pubis, 390, 1402
pubofemoral, 1404
purulent, 485
pyelitis, 660
pyelonephritis, 661
pyelonephrosis, 661
pyeloplasty, 660
pyloric sphincter, 204
pyocele, 478
pyogenic, 479, 484
pyorrhea, 480
pyorrhea, alveolaris, 489
pyorrhea salivaris, 490
pyostasis, 1378
pyothorax, 481
pyre, 971
pyrexia, 972
pyrolysis, 973
pyromaniac, 971
pyrometer, 973
pyrophilia, 1118
pyrophobia, 973
pyrosis, 972
pyrotoxin, 974

rachialgia, 1433
rachiodynia, 1434
rachiometer, 1434
rachioplegia, 1434
rachiotomy, 1433

rachischisis, 1435
rachitis, 1430, 1435
rectal, 738
rectocele, 738
rectoclysis, 739
rectocystotomy, 742
rectopexy, 746
rectoplasty, 741
rectorrhaphy, 741
rectoscope, 739
rectourethral, 742
reducible, 1522
relaxation, 1513
renal, 678
renogastric, 679
renogram, 678
renointestinal, 679
renopathy, 678
respiration, 1195
retina, 1465
retinal, 1466
retinitis, 1466
retinopexy, 1466
retinoscope, 1467
retinoscopy, 1467
retrocolic, 1007
retroflexion, 1010
retromammary, 1007
retroperitoneum, 1009
retroperitonitis, 1009
retrosternal, 1007
retroversion, 1008
Reye's syndrome, 885
rhinitis, 502
rhinolith, 508
rhinomycosis, 701
rhinoplasty, 506
rhinorrhea, 501
rhinotomy, 507

salpingectomy, 612
salpingian, 626
salpingitis, 612
salpingocele, 621
salpingo-oophorectomy, 613
salpingo-oophorocele, 614
salpingoscope, 610
salpingostomy, 611
sanguinal, 1241
sarcoma, 1279, 1348
scapular, 1413

schistocyte, 1381
schistoglossia, 1381
schistosoma, 1383
schistosomiasis, 1383
schistothorax, 1381
schizocyte, 1380
schizophasia, 1380
schizophrenia, 1380
sclera, 1452, 1455
scleral, 1455
sclerectomy, 1455
scleroiritis, 1458
sclerosis, 565
sclerostomy, 1455
scoliosis, 1234
semicomatose, 1230
semiconscious, 1228
sensitivity, 1517
sepsis, 1170
septic, 1171
septicemia, 1172
septopyemia, 1172
serous, 1519
sinister, 1318
sinistrad, 1319
sinistral, 1320
sinistrocardia, 1320
sinistrocerebral, 1320
sinistromanual, 1321
sinistropedal, 1321
spasm, 564
spermatoblast, 583
spermatocyst, 584
spermatogenesis, 582
spermatoid, 584
spermatolysis, 583
spermatopathy, 584
spermatozoa, 582
spermatozoon, 630
splenalgia, 757
splenectomy, 755
splenic, 758
splenomegaly, 755
splenopathy, 756
splenopexy, 756
splenoptosis, 755
splenorrhagia, 756
splenorrhaphy, 756
spondylitis, 1430
staphylectomy, 476
staphylitis, 475
staphylococci, 465, 469

Staphylococcus pyogenes,
  467
staphyloplasty, 474
stasis, 953, 1375
sternal, 1408
sternalgia, 1408
sternocostal, 1407
sternodynia, 1408
sternopericardial, 1407
sternum, 1406
stomatalgia, 713
stomatitis, 712
stomatomycosis, 714
stomatopathy, 714
stomatoplasty, 712
stomatorrhagia, 713
stomatoscope, 715
streptococci, 466
subabdominal, 1159
subaural, 1159
subcostal, 1162
subpubic, 1163
substernal, 1161
superciliary, 1141
superficial, 1141
superinfection, 1141
superiority, 1141
superlethal, 1141
supernumerary, 1141
supracostal, 383
supracranial, 384, 1142
supralumbar, 381, 1142
suprapelvic, 402
suprapubic, 386, 1142, 1163
suprapubic cystotomy, 389
suprarenal, 1142
suprarenoma, 1142
suprarenopathy, 1142
suprasternal, 1161
symblepharon, 1135
symbol, 1138
symbolism, 1138
symmetric, 1137
symmetrical, 1137
symmetry, 1137
sympathectomy, 1136
sympathetic, 1136
sympathoma, 1136
sympathy, 1134
symphysis, 1135
sympodia, 1136
synarthrosis, 880

syndactylism, 875
syndrome, 882–885
synergetic, 876
syphilis, 955
syphiloid, 957
syphiloma, 957
syphilopathy, 957
syphilophobe, 956
syphilophobia, 956
syphilophyma, 956
syphilopsychosis, 956
syphilosis, 956
syphilous, 956
syphilotherapy, 956
syphilotropic, 956

tachycardia, 531
tachymeter, 533
tachyphagia, 532
tachyphasia, 784
tachypnea, 538, 680
tarsals, 1167
tenodynia, 350
tenoplasty, 350
testicles (testes), 589–591
thermal, 854
thermic, 854
thermoalgesia, 854
thermoesthesia, 854
thermogenesis, 854
thermometer, 853
thermophobia, 855
thermoplegia, 855
thoracic, 439
thoracocentesis, 441, 1277
thoracolumbar, 379
thoracometer, 401
thoracopathy, 442
thoracoplasty, 443
thoracotomy, 440
thrombectomy, 576
thromboangiitis, 575
thrombocyte, 159, 580
thrombocytopenia, 158, 581
thrombogenic, 581
thromboid, 580
thrombolymphangiitis, 578
thrombolysis, 581
thrombophlebitis, 579
thrombosis, 580
thrombus, 577